WATER

can undermine
your health
!

By N. W. WALKER
Doctor of Science

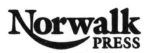

Norwalk PRESS

P O BOX 12260 / PRESCOTT AZ 86304-2260

Printed Annually Since 1974
Edited and revised 1995

ISBN: 0-89019-037-2

Manufactured in the United States of America

The drawings and sketches in this book were made by the
author solely as educational illustrations. Any resemblance to
persons living or dead is purely coincidental.

In publishing this book, it is not Dr. Walker's or the Publisher's
intent to diagnose or prescribe, but only to inform the reader.
Dr. Walker recommends the reader contact a professional doctor
specializing in the appropriate subject.

CONTENTS:

FOREWORD

Oftentimes learning the truth can be a frightening experience, but learning the answers can give new hope. Dr. Norman Walker has written many books on health over the past forty years — always with truth, conviction and, above all, *hope* that we can all live better, healthier lives.

Dr. Walker's newest book, *WATER CAN UNDERMINE YOUR HEALTH,* follows the tradition of his other books. It is written for the person who is concerned, even frightened, about the water we drink — how it affects our health, and how to avoid the problems that polluted water can create.

WATER CAN UNDERMINE YOUR HEALTH is the layman's guide to understanding and solving one of our most important health problems. Read Dr. Walker's latest book with an open mind and an eye toward better health.

Editors note: The 1995 edition contains the following additional information:

• Chapter 27: The Kidneys . . . from *Become Younger* by Dr. Walker

• Chapter 28: How Safe Is Your Drinking Water

• Chapter 29: Dr. Walker's Program to a Healthier More Vibrant Life

• ADDENDUM: A Summary of Reference Material - from which general information regarding our water supply has been gathered.

Carolyn Hoffmann, Editor

FROM THE DESK OF
DR. NORMAN WALKER . . .

In my experience of over half a century of research and observation — like many others — I have become convinced that the root or cause of nearly every ailment which afflicts the human body may be traced to the retention of waste matter in the system, and to malnutrition. We can eat many meals a day, and still be starved for lack of essential LIVE vital elements in our food.

Malnutrition results from feeding the body food which has been heated or processed to such a degree that the life of the atoms and molecules composing such food is extinct. Dead atoms and dead molecules cannot rejuvenate nor regenerate the cells in the body. Such food results in cell starvation and this in turn causes sickness and disease.

Fundamentally, it is nothing short of miraculous that people can even exist as long as they do on the kind of food so prevalent in the meals of today. Their existence cannot be attributed to the food they eat, but rather to their living in spite of the kind of food they eat.

As sickness and disease may be attributed to malnutrition, then the answer to this problem, quite naturally, would be to cleanse the system of the accumulation of waste that may be the cause of prolonging the ailment, and nourishing it with the most VITAL foods available in order to re-establish and build up that natural state of well-being that we have been taught to consider as our birthright.

N.W. Walker, D. Sc.

You don't need to relate your health to your age! For more than 100 years, Norman W. Walker, Ph.D., proved through research that well-being and long life can go hand-in-hand. Modern day nutritionists and medical researchers are just now discovering the truths which Dr. Walker has known and, expounded throughout the twentieth century. Dr. Walker himself was living proof that a longer, healthier life may be achieved through proper diet, mental soundness, and intelligent body care. Every year we read about a new fad diet, a "cure-all" drug, a food supplement, or a revolutionary exercise program that will save our lives. The Dr. Walker program is unique in that it doesn't use the promotional words, "miracle, fad, or revolutionary" ....it doesn't need them!

Dr. Walker's contributions to our living longer, healthier lives began before the turn of the century in London, where as a young man he became seriously ill from over-work. Unable to accept the idea of ill health or a sick body, Dr. Walker cured himself. Since that time, he spent the balance of his life searching man's ability to extend life and achieve freedom from disease.

In 1910, Dr. Walker established the Norwalk Laboratory of Nutritional Chemistry and Scientific Research in New York, and thus began his important contributions to a longer, more active form of living. Among his great contributions, was the discovery of the therapeutic, value of fresh vegetable juices, and in 1930 the development of the Triturator Juicer.

We believe Dr. Walker was one of the world's leading nutritionist; his unique contribution are all available to you through his books.

Chapter 1
IS THE PROBLEM REALLY SERIOUS?

Get the Doctor-Quick!
Father is having a heart attack!

When this happens, you sit up and take notice, if you have any sense. Is a heart attack a serious problem?

Is coronary thrombosis, obstruction of your arteries, a serious problem?

Is atherosclerosis, that gummy substance that slows down the blood circulation in your blood vessels until it is too late to do anything about it, a serious problem?

When the doctor arrived he took the patient's pulse, got out his stethoscope and checked the circulation of the blood. Yes, indeed, it was a preventable heart attack. It was caused by an "arterial occlusion", which, in plain language, means an obstruction of the blood vessels.

What on earth could possibly get into the arteries or into any blood vessel and cause an obstruction that could so easily result in a fatal heart attack?

Simply indigestible residue - mostly minerals from water.

The answer is simple if you will consider the processes by which the digestive system handles everything that you put in your mouth and swallow.

Look at my sketch of the digestive system which accompanies this chapter. When food or liquid has been swallowed, it travels through the stomach and in a short time enters the small intestine.

There are between 20 and 25 feet of small intestine. Everything you have swallowed must pass through it and it is either transferred to the liver for distribution into the system, or, if unable to be disintegrated it is passed on into the large intestine or colon.

Lime (calcium) is in the water, but you can't see it!

Liquids pass readily through the microscopic blood vessels in the wall of the small intestine. Whatever the liquid contains in colloidal form goes along with the liquid right into the liver. (Colloid is any substance in such a fine state of particles that it would take from 50,000,000 to 125,000,000 particles to measure one inch!) Along with the water many minerals like calcium (lime), magnesium, etc. would enter the liver.

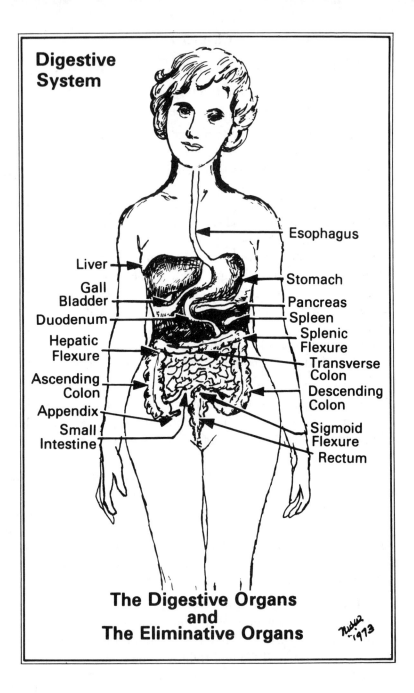

Digestive System

Esophagus

Liver

Stomach

Gall Bladder

Pancreas

Duodenum

Spleen

Hepatic Flexure

Splenic Flexure

Ascending Colon

Transverse Colon

Appendix

Descending Colon

Small Intestine

Sigmoid Flexure

Rectum

The Digestive Organs and The Eliminative Organs

Chapter 2

WHAT HAPPENS TO THE MINERALS IN THE WATER?

Hydrogen and oxygen together form the water molecule. Any other form of liquid with additional components are broken down and cleared away by the liver.

Water containing nothing but hydrogen and oxygen is pure water, and this is the only kind of water which the blood and the lymph can use in their work. Both the blood and the lymph require pure water to assist them in their functions.

Distilled Water is the purest water you can have.

Whatever mineral and chemical elements were present in the water when it first reaches the liver, are segregated by the anatomizing processes in the liver and either passed on into the blood stream or are stored away as reserve material. The liver has no selective ability to determine whether any item which comes to it is *"alive"* or inactive, whether it is constructive or detrimental.

Natural water, by which we will classify all waters that come from springs, wells, rivers and lakes, and from the faucet, is replete with mineral elements which it has collected from being in contact with earth, soil and rocks.

All the minerals in the human body — and the body is composed of minerals — are the same as the minerals of which the earth is composed. There is a vast difference between the minerals in the human body and those in the earth, not in kind or quality, but in the vitality of those which compose the human anatomy, vitality — or life — which is lacking in the earth minerals.

The body is composed of tiny microscopic cells made up of live mineral atoms. The kind, quality and variety of the mineral elements vary with each group of cells, in accordance with the functions and activities called for to carry on the cell's allotted tasks.

**Your cells need food they can swallow —
without choking to death!**

These cells MUST be furnished the mineral nourishment they need, in order to accomplish their work. Minerals which a cell or a group of cells cannot use, will only interfere with the cells function.

3

Minerals larger than those of in colloidal size particles would, figuratively speaking, choke the cells to death!

The minerals in NATURAL WATERS are gross and lifeless, and of a kind and quality which are incompatible with the cells' needs. The cells therefore reject them. In due course this rejection leaves a surprising accumulation of discarded minerals in our body.

Distilled Water leaches out ONLY unusable lime, etc.

Distilled water has an inherent ability to work much like that of a magnet. It can pick up these rejected and discarded minerals, and with the assistance of the blood and lymphatic stream, transport them to the kidneys for elimination from the system.

It is this kind of mineral elimination that is erroneously referred to as leaching. The expression that Distilled Water leaches minerals from the body is entirely inaccurate. It does not leach minerals out of the body, it collects and removes minerals which have been rejected by the cells of the body and are therefore debris, obstructing the normal functions of the system.

As a matter of fact, try drinking nothing but Distilled Water for two or three weeks. Have a urinalysis made before you start and see if you will not be astonished at the mineral sediments in the urine after a mere three weeks! There is no substitute for experience.

The accumulation of minerals in the body, from drinking Natural Waters, and the elimination of rejected minerals as a result of drinking Distilled Water is conclusive evidence of the use and value of Distilled Water for drinking and for food preparation purposes.

Vegetable Juice of carrot, beet and cucumber is a marvelous kidney cleanser.

For more than half a century we have seen the sediment in the urine of people who used to drink lots of Natural Waters. It was amazing! Fresh raw vegetable juices ARE live organic water in which the mineral elements are beautifully balanced for the nourishment of the cells of the body and for the cleansing of debris from the system. If you are not very familiar with the use of vegetable juices, study my book FRESH VEGETABLE AND FRUIT JUICES What's Missing In Your Body? (You will find it listed at the end of this book.) When the vegetable juices are raw and fresh, the water they contain is actually Distilled Water, distilled by Nature, and they contain exactly what the body needs, the finest quality of nourishment.

Distilled Water sweeps out calcified deposits — so to speak.

There is neither water nor any other liquid which can "leach" minerals out of the cells and tissues of the body, once such minerals, as organic elements, have become an integral part of the body. It is only inorganic minerals rejected by the cells and tissues of the body which, if not evacuated, can cause arterial obstructions and even more serious damage. These are the minerals which must be removed and which Distilled Water is able to collect.

What Minerals DOES the body need?

It is not intended that we should furnish the body with the minerals it must have for regeneration and replenishment, by means of the Natural Waters. The minerals which the cells of the body will use for constructive purposes must come from the raw food we eat. The only live food, food replete with enzymes, which is intended for the nourishment of man is obtained from fresh raw vegetables, fruits, herbs, nuts and seeds.

What is the principal CAUSE of most sickness and disease?

Barring accidents, the principal cause for human afflictions, except those resulting from tension and emotional disturbances, can only come from the failure to properly nourish the body. At the same time strict attention must be paid to the removal of all obstructions which interfere with the activity of the blood stream. It is equally essential to insure the regular emptying of the waste matter from the colon and from other eliminative organs.

Chapter 3
CONSTITUTION OF THE HUMAN BODY

Our dissertation on the merits and demerits of DISTILLED WATER is concerned solely with the health aspect of the arguments in favor of or against the use of either Distilled Water or of the Natural Water for drinking and for food preparation purposes.

What does concern us is the eventual effect of the use of water on the health, well-being and longevity of the individual.

Prepare for the Sunset Years of Your life!

Our particular interest is on the long range outcome of the continuous use of water for drinking and for food preparation purposes. What happens to you this week or next can be taken care of in the natural course of events.

What overtakes you 30, 50 or 70 years hence may come into the class of an irreversible affliction.

If, in the Sunset of Your life you should become crippled or otherwise incapacitated as a result of the accumulation of waste substances in your system, THAT is what we are concerned with NOW.

Know yourself - you have to live with YOU!

So, become acquainted with the cells in your body, those infinitely microscopic specks of life that constitute your anatomy, the cells that build, compose and constitute the tissues out of which every part of your system is constructed.

Your body is composed of billions upon billions of these tiny, infinitely small specks of life known as cells.

Just as a baby is fed by bottle or by the teaspoonful, because larger amounts of food could not be handled, so it is with the tiny cells in your system. The food of these cells consists of extremely minute particles of the minerals required for their activities, as minute as from one-millionth to 100-millionth part of a grain. Grosser particles they cannot utilize. (Note: There are about 440 grains to the ounce. 1-millionth part of a grain is, therefore, approximately 440-millionth parts of an ounce and 100-millionth part of a grain equals approximately 44-thousand-millionth part of one ounce. If you can visualize such microscopic amounts you are truly a wizard.)

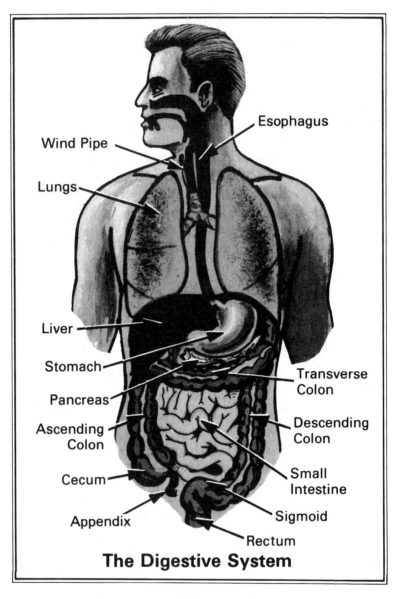

The Digestive System

Your lungs - Take care of them.
You can't buy new ones!

When you can't get oxygen in your lungs, it's *Finis! - The End!*
Oxygen is, without exception, the most important, vital requirement
of your life. Oxygen is collected from the air you breathe through
your lungs. It is transported from the lungs by the blood to the cells.

Any interference with the function of your lungs means a corresponding drain on the vitality of the years ahead.

Upon receipt of the oxygen, the cells are able to convert minerals into the organic pattern which forms the matrix for the many and varied parts of the anatomy, such as the muscles, nerves, membranes, connective tissues, etc.

The most constructive minerals are those which are contained in the raw vegetables, fruits, herbs, nuts and seeds. These minerals are an integral part of the live organic water of the juices of these natural raw products. This "vegetation" water (i.e. the juices) is the result of the distillation by plant process, of moisture from the atmosphere and from the water obtained from the ground, and is replete with enzymes, the natural LIFE principle. It is truly DISTILLED WATER.

Chapter 4

THERE ARE MINERALS
AND MINERALS; LEACH WHICH?

The minerals in the Natural Waters are inactive. They do not contain enzymes, the essence of life. Nature has made a provision to instill life into these mineral elements by means of the development of the growth and maturity of plants. In the course of the plant's growth the roots collect minerals from the earth, convert them into live organic elements and absorb them into the stem, the leaves, the seeds, and the flower and fruit.

It is natural that the use of fresh raw vegetable and fruit juices should furnish the cells and tissues of the body with the finest kind and quality of nourishment in the form of ultra-microscopic minerals replete with enzymes.

The true nectar for your best friends —
the cells of your body!

The body cells use *these* live organic minerals avidly. The processes of replenishment and regeneration by means of such nourishment enable the body to avoid and overcome the afflictions caused by the lack of such nourishment that has plagued generation after generation, shortening man's life-span.

To help retard the processes of premature and decrepit old age it is essential that the body be nourished with live foods in abundance, besides drinking plenty of Distilled Water daily.

To enable the cells of the body to obtain their mineral nourishment the fastest and the most efficient way is by the use of fresh raw vegetable and fruit juices. I need not expound here on this subject of Juice Therapy and Nutrition as I have covered this matter extensively and in great detail in my two books FRESH VEGETABLE AND FRUIT JUICES, What's Missing In Your Body? and GUIDE TO DIET & SALAD which are listed at the end of this book.

The foundation of knowledge is laid by reading.
Wisdom from its application.

A study of the contents of these books will, I am sure, if put into practice, convince the most skeptic that, while the human system needs minerals in its nourishment, emphasis should center first and foremost on the selection of nourishment in relation to the needs of the body.

The needs to satisfy the appetite is a different matter. Appetite is the craving of the mind, whereas hunger is the call of the cells of the body for nourishment.

Cultivate hunger. Banish appetites.

You can satisfy your appetite with whatever your craving dictates. In that case the kind and nature of the minerals in what you eat and drink is of little consequence, if you don't care. When satisfaction is the result of eating and drinking what is incompatible for the welfare of your body, you are the victim of your cravings. Whatever afflictions perplex and plague you eventually will be more no less a result of the water and foods you have consumed over your lifetime.

When you have learned to control your appetites and your cravings, and center your choice of food on what will regenerate and replenish your system, you will be giving the cells and tissues of your body the live mineral elements they need. They, in turn, will reward you with health, energy, vigor, vitality and a longer life. But you must keep your colon cleaned out. The accumulation of corruption in the colon does more damage than most people realize.

Chapter 5

NATURAL WATERS PLAGUE THE BLOODSTREAM

If you REALLY want to know the facts about the deposit of calcium, magnesium and other minerals in the veins and arteries of your body from using Natural Waters, you simply MUST know something about the blood and the blood vessels in your system.

Without some factual knowledge on the subject what kind of an opinion can you form? How can you possibly determine whether YOU will use Natural Water - and suffer the consequences, or use DISTILLED WATER - and be safe?

The contents of your blood:

Your blood is composed of 78% by volume, of fluid, and 90% , yes, ninety percent, of the fluid is PURE DISTILLED WATER, (pure H_2O) 8% to 9% content is protein and less than 1% consists of substances which the blood has picked up in the course of its travels throughout your body. These substances consist of unusable minerals such as calcium, magnesium, etc., amino acids, fats, urea, uric acid, ammonia salts and many others.

You only have about 5 Quarts of blood in your system!

Your entire body contains only about 5 quarts of blood and each tiny drop of blood is composed of more than 3,000,000 blood cells. Every cell in your body is composed of millions of atoms of mineral elements.

Every drop of your blood flows through your heart more than 103,000 times every 24 hours.

The small total volume of 5 quarts of your blood, passing through your heart, will have equaled about 164,000,000 quarts of blood, equal to some 300,000,000 pounds of blood during a mere 70-year lifespan.

No pump in the world equals Your Heart!

No pumping mechanism was ever devised by man to do the work your heart does and to take the punishment that your heart gets, yet the size of your heart is only about the size of your clenched fist. It measures approximately 4¾ inches in length, 3½ inches in width and is about 2¼ inches thick. It is given to you as a literal birthday present and is intended to last for centuries if it could only get the proper nourishment and attention.

Chapter 6

MINERALS CAN ACCUMULATE DANGEROUSLY!

Will You drink 4500 gallons of Spring water?

With this fantastic picture about your heart and your blood, realize that a person drinking about two pints of Natural Water a day, besides other beverages, will have had more than 4,500 gallons of water pass through his body during the 70-year lifespan.

Do You want 300 pounds of lime to pass through Your body?

The inorganic mineral elements which were contained in that water, and which the cells could not use, will have been deposited in the body, mostly in the veins, arteries, muscles and joints, and added all up, may have totalled between 200 and 300 pounds during the 70 years! These minerals would consist of the calcium (lime), magnesium, and other mineral elements. Naturally they did not all stay in the body.

Fortunately, most of these minerals were collected by the blood, lymph and water in the system, and passed out through the excretory channels. Who could ever tell how much of it remained in the veins and arteries, in the muscles and joints? Only premature old age and a crippled and afflicted body could give the answer.

The "Father who had a stroke" maybe did!

Turn to the "father who had a stroke" on the first chapter of this book. Never forget that, but remember that millions of people are constantly drinking natural water, and continue to live. Will they die prematurely?

The largest artery in the body, the aorta, measures about one inch in diameter, but that is no criterion when you realize the size and number of the microscopic capillaries which are spread throughout the entire anatomy.

The tiny capillaries in your body form a network which, if spread out on the ground, would cover an area of about 1½ acres. That's about 63,000 square feet. If all these tiny capillaries were placed end to end, they would make a microscopic tube about 60 miles in length. How many of these would get clogged up with the calcium, magnesium and other minerals in Natural Waters?

Chapter 7

DANGER FROM WATER - OLD AS THE HILLS

Do you for a moment think that the dangers of drinking Natural Waters is a present-day discovery, a fad? You are wrong!

Way back, in 1845 - that's one hundred and twenty eight years ago as of this year, while I am typing this manuscript - Mr. Abel Haywood lectured, taught, preached, wrote and admonished people of the fatal dangers lurking in all Natural Waters.

Life CAN be prolonged!

He wrote a dissertation on the subject, in England, in which he stated:

"Let it not be said that the life of man cannot be prolonged to many times the present period of his existence, because it is not so, . . . The common reasoning adopted by the world has been sufficient to bring ridicule, and even punishment and death, upon those who have ventured to propose anything out of the common path, even though it has ultimately been the source of great delight to the persecutors themselves."

The following is extracted from Mr. Haywood's booklet: (The headings are mine.)

What makes people stiff

"The solid earthy matter which by gradual accumulation in the body brings on ossification, rigidity, decrepitude and death, is principally phosphate of lime, or bone matter, carbonate of lime, or common chalk; and sulphate lime, or Plaster of Paris, with occasionally magnesia and other earthy substances.

Old age stiffness begins in INFANCY!

"We have seen that a process of consolidation begins at the earliest period of existence, and continues without interruption until the body is changed from a comparatively fluid, elastic and energetic state, to a solid, earthy, rigid, inactive condition which terminates in death. That infancy, childhood, youth, manhood, old age, decrepitude, are but so many different conditions of the body between old age and youth, is the greater density, toughness and rigidity, and the greater proportion of calcareous earthy matter which enters into its composition.

Where does obstruction of the arteries come from?

"The question now arises: what is the source of the calcareous earthy matter which thus accumulates in the system? It seems to be regarded as an axiom that all the solids of the body are continually built up and renewed by the blood. If so, everything which these solids contain is derived from the blood: the solids contain phosphates and carbonate of lime which are therefore derived from the blood in which these earthy substances are invariably found.

Water contents frightful to contemplate!

"Spring water contains an amount of earthy ingredients which is fearful to contemplate. It has been calculated that water of an average quality contains so much carbonate and other compounds of lime, that a person drinking an average quantity each day will, in 40 years, have taken as much into his body as would form a pillar of solid chalk or marble as large as a good sized man.

Enough minerals in Water to choke-up the body.

"So great is the amount of lime in spring water, that the quantity taken daily would alone be sufficient to choke up the system so as to bring on decrepitude and death long before we arrived at 20 years of age, were it not for the kidneys and other secreting organs throwing it off in considerable quantities.

Only a Portion of Water-minerals retained in body.

"These organs, however, only discharge a portion of this matter; for instance, supposing 10 parts to be taken during a day, 8 or 9 may be thrown out, and one or two lost somewhere in the body.

Enfeebled rigidity is progressive.

"This process continuing day after day and year after year, the solid matter at length accumulates until the activity and flexibility of childhood becomes lost in the enfeebled rigidity of what is then called (though very erroneously) "old age".

Calcium in pans and kettle!

"A familiar instance of earthy deposition and incrustation from water is observed in a common kettle or steam boiler. Every housewife knows that a vessel which is in constant use will soon become " furred-up", or plastered on the bottom and sides with a hard stony substance, 4 and 5 pounds in weight of this matter have been known to collect in 12 months.

Steam leaves Minerals behind - in kettle!

"Do not be misled by thinking that because so much lime is found in a teakettle, the water remaining after boiling it is therefore free from lime. It is true that boiling water does cause a little carbonate of lime to precipitate, but the bulk of the sediment is left from that portion of the water ONLY which is driven off by steam, or has boiled away.

Filtering the Water is useless.

"Filtering it is also of no use, for this only removes what may be floating or mechanically mixed with the water, whereas the earthy matter here spoken of is held in solution.

Clear, transparent Water is full of Minerals!

"Spring water, clear and transparent as it may appear, is nevertheless charged with a considerable amount of solid choking-up matter and is therefore unfit or at least not the best suited for internal use."

Note: The foregoing is quoted from a booklet which Mr. Abel Haywood published in England in 1845. The complete text you will find in my book VIBRANT HEALTH, The Possible Dream.

Chapter 8
COMPARE THE PAST TO THE PRESENT

If the water problem was as bad as that, way back over 128 years ago, what would Mr. Haywood have to say about our vexing water problems of this day and generation?

They had no chlorination problem in those days, nor were they plagued with the matter of fluoridation.

The industry, as recently as one century ago, was not faced with the colossal waste disposal vexation which faces our present civilization.

Today's griefs.

It is bad enough, today, to be afflicted with the specter of progressively calcified arteries which expunged thousands upon thousands in past generations. The addition of poisonous substances to the water is really an inexcusable lack of intelligence and foresight. To kill germs, virus and bacteria is one thing, but to slowly destroy a people by the use of poisonous pesticides is inexcusable.

Know what you drink.

Once water has been saturated with these noxious (if not lethal) ingredients, people who have been misinformed will drink and prepare food with it, altogether oblivious of the eventual effect on their health and lifespan.

It seems useless to try to help people who won't be helped!

There are two areas of education which are profoundly effective, as a rule. One area is to visit Old People's Homes and Sanitaria. It is truly heartbreaking to see how people have let themselves deteriorate without ever, through their whole life, realizing that they were eating their way and drinking their progression into premature decrepitude and uselessness, to say nothing of an improvident demise.

Can people be taught a lesson from these examples of human waste?

The other area for deep educational enlightenment is the study of middle-aged people lying on the table of a Mortician, waiting for the Coroner to give his verdict. Look at the vast number of obituaries of people who killed themselves through lack of knowledge of fundamental principles of nutrition, waste evacuation and control of emotions.

I have seen and studied hundreds of such people and I have learned MY lesson!

Chapter 9
SOFT DRINKS?

What's wrong with Soft Drinks?

Supposing you knew that Soft Drinks could cause your brain to disintegrate, would you drink them?

More than a million children today are afflicted with cerebral lesions and other afflictions caused by Soft Drinks!

This is not a wild assertion. This is a very important discovery which has been made by Medical Research.

By drinking beverages and eating foods which have been artificially colored and flavored, millions of school children are TODAY suffering serious ailments. These disturbances have been diagnosed as cerebral lesions, that is injury to the brain that causes sudden discharge of excessive nervous energy.

This disturbance results in difficulty to concentrate, in reading and in spelling. It also causes strange compulsive aggressive behavior.

The affliction disappears when drinks and foods artificially colored and flavored are strictly eliminated from the diet.

When children, under strict supervision, have been deprived of Soft Drinks and of all foods with artificial additives of color and flavor, the children in many cases became normal within a matter of about three weeks. On the other hand, after the ailment was conquered, it would immediately return within a matter of hours if as much as a sip or one morsel of artificially colored or flavored product was indulged in.

This problem is tremendously serious and every parent should be alerted to it. It is proof of the hazard and danger of using artificially colored and flavored products. It is usually children of normal or outstanding intelligence who are afflicted by this peril.

Adults also affected - eventually.

Adult office and factory workers consistently drinking Soft Drinks are also liable to be afflicted with similar brain or cerebral lesions. They feel a "lift" while imbibing these and even for a short while after, but such an uplift is elusive and evanescent, the letdown resulting in fatigue, poor concentration, and frequently headaches.

Distilled Water is always beneficial.

In the absence of fresh raw vegetable and fruit juices, there is no better and healthier thirst quencher than Distilled Water. Thirst is thus quenched and satisfied with greater benefit and effectiveness.

Don't overlook the danger from the calcium in the water in Soft Drinks.

While the calcium and other mineral elements present in the water of Soft Drinks may cause afflictions by obstructing the blood vessels, the ingredients used in the conversion of water into Brand Name products is far more insidious. Such ingredients in the form of artificial flavoring and coloring act much sooner than would the calcium in clogging up the system, because of their effect on the chemistry of the body.

What are these extraneous Ingredients?

Sugar is one of the most harmful ingredients used in the manufacture of Soft Drinks.

The public has been led to develop a "sweet tooth" and a taste for sugar. Consequently, in order to make the Soft Drinks saleable the manufacturers have established a standard for taste which will appeal to people of all ages, irrespective of the consequences.

What's harmful about sugar?

What a question to ask! I thought EVERYBODY knew that sugar causes irritation and weakening of the mucous membranes of the body and robs teeth, bones and blood of a great percentage of their minerals. Inflammatory diseases of the breathing and digestive organs result from the use of white and brown sugar. Diseases of the throat, nose, chest and of the skin are frequently due to the use of white and brown sugar.

When the human body is overloaded with such sugar and sugar mixtures, both in solid and in liquid form, the vitality of the body cells is afflicted and this may cause swellings and mucous discharges. Inflammatory diseases increase and are intensified in direct proportion to the amount of sugar used.

Appendicitis has to a large extent been caused by the excessive use of sugar sweetened products.

Diabetes and cancer have been traced to the excessive use of sugar, and so has poliomyelitis, an inflammation of the grey matter of the spinal cord, which causes painful crippling of the body.

All this is, in my opinion, a good and sufficient reason for classifying sugar as harmful. More about sugar presently.

Do the labels on bottles and packages mean anything to you?
Do you check the labels to see what you are buying?

Have you and your children been buying Soft Drinks in bottles or cans? Have you and your children bought those 10¢ and 25¢ envelopes to the contents of which you need only to add water to make a Soft Drink? Did you read the labels?

If the labels were marked POISON, would you buy them?

Did you ever analyze the word POISON? Here is what it means, ponder over its broad interpretation: *Any agent which, introduced into the organism may chemically produce an injurious or deadly effect. That which taints or destroys purity, to exert a baneful influence, to corrupt.* Remember this about every purchase you and your children make, of food of any and every kind, and you will not be too far wrong. Train your children to read labels.

What are the objectionable ingredients
in artificial drinks and foods?

It is incredible but true that more than 80%, that's right, more than eighty percent of the manufactured beverages and foods sold in markets and stores are compounded from chemicals using artificial colors and flavors to make them saleable.

While the human body can take a great deal of punishment and survive, it is nevertheless a very delicate organism created to be fed and maintained according to certain natural and physiological laws. When the body is properly cared for according to these laws we can expect Vibrant Health and a long and comfortable life.

When human nature allows the human element of appetite to control the individual and a person indulges in beverages and foods which are not compatible with these natural and physiological laws, the natural sequence is pain, sickness, disease and a premature old age.

We are learning from these pages, what the hazard is likely to be when we drink Natural waters which contain inorganic calcium and may eventually clog up veins and arteries.

There is a far greater hazard, in fact there is the actual danger, when chemically concocted foods and beverages are used, that a chemical reaction may cause serious disturbances in the body. The greatest danger is when the brain area is afflicted by the chemical constituents of such drinks.

The following is a partial list of artificial ingredients copied from some bottles, cans, envelopes and packages on market shelves:

Aniline Dyes: You will rarely find aniline dyes mentioned by their names. They are generally classified as "artificial coloring. Some of these dyes are very acidic and you should know at least some of the worst. While such dyes affect the body adversely, their reaction may vary in different types of people.

AMARANTH (red), BORDEAUX (brown), ORANGE I (yellow) and PONCEAU (scarlet) are all derived from compounding nitrogen and benzene. Benzene is obtained from the distillation of coal. It is used as a motor fuel, as a solvent for resins, rubber, etc., and in the manufacture of dyes. It is an ingredient in coloring beverages. As chemical compounds these dyes are harmful because they afflict the nerve system and the cerebrospinal fluid.

GUINEA GREEN (dark green) is a dye obtained by the reaction of chloroform with benzene and aluminum chloride. Chloroform has a sweetish taste. It is used as an anesthetic to put people to sleep. It produces violent gastroenteritis (inflammation of the bowel and of the stomach) and complete unconsciousness when taken alone internally. Aluminum chloride is derived from heating aluminum with chlorine. It is used in oil refineries for "cracking" oils. The effect of aluminum on the body manifests in neuralgia, loss of energy, constipation, skin troubles, nausea, loss of appetite and many other afflictions.

NAPHTHOL (yellow) is compounded by nitrogen and benzene extracted from coal and is a coal tar product. It is used in the manufacture of dyes. Coal tar products can have very serious and harmful effects on the system, Cancer is just one of the hazards.

TARTRAZINE (yellow) is obtained by the action of acetylene on diazo-methane, producing a poisonous chemical which is nevertheless used as a coloring agent in beverages and foods. This word 'poisonous" should warn and alert you.

Whenever you read "ARTIFICIAL COLORING" on a label there is no indication whatever which dyes are used for this purpose. It could be any one or a combination of these.

Artificial Flavors:

As is the case with the use of artificial colors, there are innumerable substances used to give beverages and foods or whatever the product, a flavor as nearly as possible to that of the fruit or flavor they try to imitate. The product may not have been within miles of the fruit imitated, so artificial compounds are added to make the product palatable. The following are some examples of what is used:

CARAMEL is obtained by heating sugar to more than 350°F, or molasses or glucose, with ammonia. Besides using caramel as a red-yellow coloring agent, it adds a sugary zest to the flavor. The use of caramel tends to throw the blood out of balance, causing heart trouble which is intensified by the presence of ammonia. When used in excessive amounts it can cause mental and other disorders, particularly in children.

CITRIC ACID is present in live organic form in citrus fruits, in which state it is beneficial as an alkalinizing beverage. When citric acid is made chemically, however, and used in Soft Drinks, it increases the negative acidity of the system. If the organic citric acid were used in Soft Drinks it would make the price almost prohibitive, whereas if it is made chemically its cost would be considerably cheaper. Such chemical citric acid can cause canker sores in the mouth and even ulcers in the duodenum.

Would you enjoy some Mexican Lice in your Soft Drink?

COCHINEAL is a dye consisting of the dried bodies of LICE which feed on cacti in Mexico and other parts of Central and South America. Special cacti are extensively cultivated for the express purpose of propagating the Cochineal lice. The female louse is gathered and killed by heat, then dried and pulverized. It yields a bright Castillian red. It is rarely if ever mentioned as Cochineal but may find its way in almost any product as "artificial coloring." It is also known as QUILLAJA.

Cola Drinks. Facts which imbibers should know!

COCA is a South American and African nut containing 2% caffeine, theobromine and tannin. It is analogous to coffee. In normal doses it stimulates the brain causing nervous restlessness and wakefulness. In larger doses it produces insomnia, paralysis of the heart muscles, convulsions, delirium, and other afflictions.

COLA is a plant grown throughout South America and in India. It is the derivative of cocaine, causing stimulation of the brain, resulting in normal sex desires being inhibited, it increases heart action and the irritability of the nerves, followed by mental, moral and muscular depression. It deadens the sensation of hunger and thirst temporarily but greatly increases these when the effects wear off. It gives a temporary sense of hilarity and well-being. Eventually the individual may look haggard and worn-out.

CORN STARCH is the product of milling corn with a final washing in caustic soda. In the process, the hull and the germ (the germ is the living substance, the embryo or life of the seeds in plants) are removed. It is then steeped in a solution of sulphuric dioxide gas to prevent fermentation.

The oil is then extracted and the residue of the germ is made into cakes for fattening cattle and sheep. The starch granules, in their coarse state, are used as cattle feed while the rest of the granules which form a white flour are cleaned with caustic soda and sold for human consumption. Corn starch appears smooth, fluffy and white but carries with it a most noxious odor that flows quite liberally from this highly caustic substance. As you probably know, caustic soda is commonly used in bleaching, making soap and refining industrial oils. The digestion of Corn Starch has no constructive purpose while, on the other hand, whether used as a starch or in beverages, it tends to clog up the fine filtering tissues of the connective tissues, veins and arteries.

CORN SYRUP is a transparent thick glucose obtained from corn starch by heating the starch with acids which prevents its crystallizing. It is used as a cheap sweetening agent. Corn syrup quickly turns into alcohol in the digestive system and may have the tendency to dissolve fat soluble Vitamins in the body. It also has the tendency to interfere with the functions of the pancreas, particularly if there is a tendency to diabetes.

DEXTROSE is a natural sugar present in animal and plant tissues, but DEXTRIN is made commercially by the decomposition of starch by the action of acids. Mixed with iodine it yields a red color. It is used in the manufacture of adhesives, for sizing, as a substitute for gums, in making Soft Drinks, and in beer. Obviously such a product can readily cause many types of ailments and physical and mental disturbances when their end product in digestion reaches the brain area, and interferes with the normal functions of the nerves and muscles and of the cerebrospinal fluid.

GLUCOSE occurs in the digestion of carbohydrates, in Nature, but commercially it is made by heating starch (mainly corn starch) with acid in order to make a cheap corn syrup used in Soft Drinks.

POTASSIUM CHLORIDE occurs in animal and plant fluids but when used in industry it is made commercially as a fertilizer and for use in Soft Drinks.

POTASSIUM PHOSPHATE is an acid component for fertilizers and is used in Soft Drinks with carbonated waters to effervesce or "fizz" the beverage.

SODIUM CITRATE is used as a prescription for certain genitourinary diseases. It is also used in Soft Drinks as an additive to give them the citric acid "zip".

SACCHARIN is manufactured on a large scale from coal tar and formed by dehydrating saccharinic acid. While it is from 300 to 500 times sweeter than cane sugar, it has no food value whatever. On the contrary, like every coal tar product, it has a definite acid reaction on the system. Any inorganic acid reaction on the system has a detrimental effect on the Endocrine Gland functions of the body.

SODIUM PHOSPHATE occurs in the blood and in the urine. It is made artificially as a dye coloring agent and is used in weighting silk. It is also used as artificial coloring for Soft Drinks. Like all chemically manufactured substances, sodium phosphate interferes with the normal smooth functions of the Endocrine Glands throwing the body functions out of balance.

SALT used in Soft Drinks is the same as table salt. Such salt, whatever it has been obtained from, is heated at tremendously high temperatures to prevent its being affected by moisture so it will pour from the saltshaker. Tumors and cancer have been known to result from the use of salt. In fact when patients afflicted with tumors resumed the use of salt after foregoing the use of it for some time, the size of the tumor grew in size perceptibly. In countries where the consumption of foods are used which have been saturated in salt, cancer has been noticeably on the increase.

The abundant use of salt can readily cause high blood pressure and hypertension, heart ailments and kidney trouble.

An excessive use of salt can cause ear and sinus trouble and it has been a contributing factor in nervous tension, rheumatism and hives.

SUGAR. We gave a brief reference to sugar early in our dissertation on the subject of Soft Drinks, but I would feel remiss, if in my exploitation of this subject of sugar, I failed to emphasize the importance of avoiding the use of all white and brown sugar for the sake of attaining Vibrant Health. Near the conclusion of the subject of Soft Drinks, therefore, I want to add more emphasis on the detrimental effects of sugar on the body.

Unquestionably, sugar is very important in the function of metabolism. There is always sugar present in the blood stream, which is known as blood sugar, and this is an essential component of the human system. White sugar, however, is no more like blood sugar than a horsechestnut is like a chestnut horse. This applies also to the comparison of white and brown sugar with honey and with the sugar in fresh fruits.

Never be deceived by the expression used in sugar advertisements as PURE SUGAR. This expression, Pure Sugar, in this case means that everything of nutritional value has been removed from the product, leaving a lifeless, useless substance which, when ingested, rushes through the stomach to become alcohol even before the liver has a chance to work on it.

Why do supposedly intelligent people imbibe Soft Drinks?

This question of why people imbibe Soft Drinks, has puzzled me for a very long time. Would it be a quirk in the human mind that would fail to cause a person to be individualistic and abstain from putting something in their body which would cause eventual suffering? Or could it be that they are not aware of the ultimate destruction which they are building up in their body?

Diabetes is a notorious example of the use of white sugar in food products and in beverages.

Coronary thrombosis, the disease resulting from the clogging up of veins and arteries, is very frequently the result of using too much sugar in ANY form.

Mothers should train and educate their babies and their children, as they are growing up, to avoid sweet foods and beverages that have been flavored or sweetened with white or brown sugar or artificially sweetened and flavored, pointing out to them the eventual dangers which will afflict them the rest of their lives. Surely mothers are definitely interested in the health and welfare, and the health and longevity of their offspring. White and brown sugar can reduce the life span of people by as much as fifteen percent.

Is it worth indulging a sweet tooth, with sugar? I say NO!

Read the Labels on everything You buy — Be Aware — Learn to Discriminate.

Chapter 10

WHAT EVIL LURKS IN A KEG OF BEER?

Beer is hypnotic.

Beer has a peculiar hypnotic fascination for nearly every one who drinks beer habitually. The average alcohol content of beer ranges only between 3% and 5%. It is generally assumed that, because of the low alcohol content, beer is an innocuous beverage. This is a very deceptive assumption because, actually, beer gives a long-range degenerative reaction.

Alcohol is bad!

Alcohol is the only substance which will pass straight through the walls of the stomach, and is picked up by the blood and carried directly to the areas of the brain. That is the reason why one's actions are unpredictable once an alcoholic drink has slipped down the throat.

The low alcoholic content of beer does not have the immediate reaction like that of a cocktail or of drinking straight potions like whisky, vodka, champagne and the like.

Beer works more slowly.

The alcohol in beer is much more subtle in its harmful effects. The period which elapses between drinking a glass of beer as a stimulant and its reaction on the body involves the element of time because of the three phases in which the reaction takes effect.

Beer seduces the senses.

In the first place, there is the period of excitement and of entrancement which gratifies and seduces the sense organs and transmits the stimulation to the nerve centers.

Beer excites the midriff.

In the second place, the low alcoholic content is just enough to create an excited activity in the midriff, the center of the system, the region of the solar plexus. This activity is insidiously dangerous because there is nothing to counteract it nor to counterbalance it. Frequently small doses of any substance turn out to be far more powerful than massive doses.

For example: Calcium-sulphate (Plaster of Paris) if swallowed in large amounts like a tablespoonful or a cupful at a time, will clog up the entire digestive system in a matter of minutes or hours. When

Calcium-sulphate, as a Biochemic cell-salt, is taken in fractional amounts of 5-millionths part of a grain, it is beneficial and has effectively banished boils, abscesses, lung trouble, etc.

Beer can cause serious ailments.

In the third place, hops in the beer has an unhealthy reaction on the system.

The hops used in making beer (Humulus Lupulus) are used for the purpose of adding flavor and an extra "zip". Not many people, apparently, are aware of the noxious effect of hops on health. The damage which results from the calcium and other mineral elements in the water as a clogging medium interferes with the blood circulation and is aggravated by the evanescent uplift of the low alcoholic content of the beer.

From a health standpoint, while hops is used medicinally as a tonic and a stimulant, it affects the nerves, creating a loss of sensation. Hops also have a hypnotic effect and can cause delirium tremors, or specifically a violent state of delirium induced by the alcohol itself. Other afflictions resulting from the use of hops can be hysteria, nervous insomnia, dyspepsia, rheumatism, and irritation of the bladder.

Long range damage by beer.

This comparison gives you a mental picture of what is meant by the long-range effect of doses of alcohol in minute quantities. The effects of drinking beer may continue for some hours, until the nerves carry the stimulating impulses away from the midriff towards the outward or peripheral or motor nerve centers. Once there, the person's actions and functions are likely to be interfered with to a more or less degree of severity.

Degeneration of the kidneys and the brain.

These conclusions are based on the study of the heaviest beer-drinking people in the civilized world, the Germans, the British, Australians and Americans. These various and diverse studies follow a very close pattern, enough to form a fairly dependable conclusion. It indicates the closeness with which the eventual endproduct effect of the digestion of beer can cause degeneration of the kidneys and of the cerebral or brain areas.

They were drinking beer 6000 years ago!

According to archeological discoveries, beer made from cereals has been recognized as used for some 6000 years. It was made from the fermentation of the cereals to obtain the alcoholic effect. It is recorded that about 5000 years ago, in the year 3000 B.C., in Egypt, four types of beer were made from grains grown in that country. The Pharaohs paid their peasants 4 loaves of bread and 2 jugs of beer as recompense for their labor, instead of paying them money.

Rameses 3rd of Egypt gave beer to his gods!

Somewhat more recently, in 1200 B.C. the Pharaoh Rameses boasted of having contributed 465,000 jugs of beer to his pagan deities.

Fermented cereals - beer.

Through the centuries cereals were grown to a great extent for making beer by the process of fermentation. Barley, wheat and oats were the most commonly used. Hops were added occasionally 40 to 50 centuries ago.

Blame your beer for your bladder and kidney trouble!

As a matter of fact, bladder and kidney troubles are most prolific in the civilized countries above mentioned, the countries in which beer consumption is the highest.

Manufactured each year, Billions of gallons of beer!

The production of beer in the United States of America exceeds 3,875,000,000, yes, more than 3¾ BILLION gallons a year. In England it is more than 750,000,000 gallons!

If you drink beer, don't ever say:
I don't drink enough to do any harm. It's a lie!

Quite naturally, most people who drink beer claim that they don't drink enough beer to cause their health to be seriously affected.

This is self-deception. Because affliction does not overtake the beer drinker within a day or two, tnevertheless the fact remains that ailments which may eventually appear may not be considered nor will they be traced to their real cause. Furthermore, no thought is given to the calcium and magnesium incrustations which may remain in the body from drinking the water from which the beer was made.

They add Gypsum to the water in
making beer-why not cement?

Beer making requires such hard water that the manufacturers frequently have to add as much as 35 times more minerals than are present in the water supply, using vast quantities of GYPSUM. Gypsum is a calcium-sulphate used for making Plaster of Paris. The purpose of this is to increase the calcium content of the water. Isn't that NICE? And people drink beer without a thought of the Plaster of Paris they are drinking, which eventually may block their arteries.

This knowledge about beer is a must, for everyone who cares.

I would feel guilty of the sin of omission if I failed to include in this book this long dissertation about one of the most common habits which men and women are addicted to - drinking beer on any and every occasion. Far be it from me to attempt to dissuade anyone from drinking beer, if he has a mind to do so. After reading this chapter one can do as he pleases. My conscience is clear.

Study the accompanying illustration of beer damage!

Let us take a few minutes to look into the Kidneys:

So many people seem to think that the kidneys are merely a receptacle for liquids with some mysterious automatically controlled relief valves. Not so! A section cut across through the kidney reveals a vast number of tiny blood vessels, in groups, called glomureli. These glomureli form continuous tubes which, at the entrance in which the blood flows, is larger than that through which it passes out. This constriction at the outlet causes a high degree of pressure to form continually. The purpose of this is to enable the blood to disgorge from its contents the liquids and substances which are to be excreted. These are mineral salts and other contents of the water, such as urea, uric acid, etc. Under such pressure these extraneous substances pass into the funnel shaped expansion at the upper end of the ureter, the tube which leads liquids out of the kidneys.

Ah! Here come the kidney stones!

You should be able to figure out how simply, under these circumstances, the fine particles of calcium and other unusable substances and minerals, start clogging up these extremely fine passages. This is how and where kidney stones are formed, and kidney stones are frequently the first step in the development of urinary afflictions.

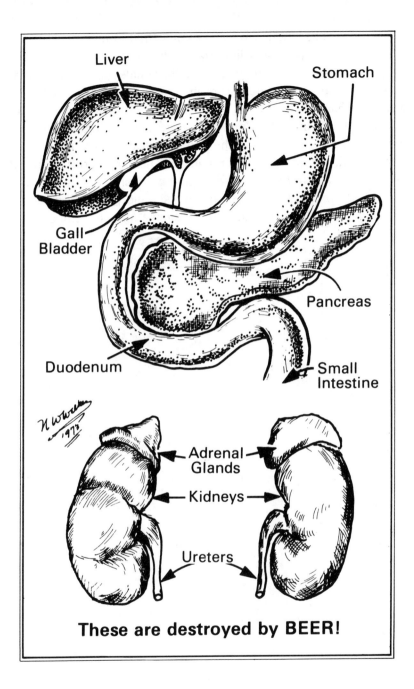

Liver

Stomach

Gall Bladder

Pancreas

Duodenum

Small Intestine

Adrenal Glands

Kidneys

Ureters

These are destroyed by BEER!

The calcium which reaches the kidneys
is exactly like that in the kettle.

Again I must call your attention to the results seen in the bottom of the kettle in which water has been boiled repeatedly, whether the water was hard or soft water. The sediment collected on the bottom of such kitchen utensils is mute evidence of the calcium and other minerals left as residue, after the water, as steam, has left the kettle. Similar mineral residues pass through the veins and arteries as a result of drinking water from faucets, wells, springs, rivers etc. Heart attacks, coronary thrombosis, arthritis, rheumatism and many other painful afflictions can be traced to such residue remaining in the body.

Chapter 11

WINE AND LIQUOR?

Can't I drink a glass of wine?

Wines and liquors have no place in this dissertation, strictly speaking, because no water is used in their manufacture.

Some pertinent remarks on the damages caused by alcohol, which are not generally known, may not be entirely out of place here, as these beverages are responsible for more broken homes, more accidents, more fatalities, more crime, more delinquency . . . in fact more of everything that is evil, disrupting and immoral than any other factor in civilization.

The average alcoholic content of wines is in the neighborhood of 15%. "Hard liquor" contains a disastrously high percentage of alcohol which causes, in the drinker, a speedy impetus to mental and physical behavior which is inverse to his natural self.

Alcohol's First Stop — The Brain!

The most damaging alcoholic evil is the affliction which these beverages cause to the human brain. Alcohol is the only substance which can pass through the walls of the stomach directly into the bloodstream. It is picked up by the blood and transported quickly to the brain areas. The most important and the most vital, sensitive impulses, functions and activities are generated in the brain.

Do You want to dissolve your brain in Alcohol?

There are many cells in the human body which are composed of elements which are either only soluble in alcohol or are dangerously afflicted by it. As an example, consider the crystalline sugar analogous to glucose, which is present in the brain tissues and is known as Cerebrose. This substance is quickly affected by alcohol. It is closely involved in the cerebrospinal fluid which, through the hypothalamus in the midbrain regulates the eyeballs, the ears and the individuals equilibrium or balance. You can readily see where bleary-eyes, uncertain hearing, and a wobbly walk are indicative of having indulged in alcohol. When this Cerebrose substance dissolves and appears in the urine it indicates the serious condition known as cerebral diabetes.

Of all the beverages best left alone, alcoholic beverages are Number ONE.

Chapter 12

SEA WATER

Don't drink it!

Sea Water is not, under any circumstances, intended to be used for drinking purposes. Nor can the water from inland salt water lakes be used as a beverage.

The very high volume of sodium-chloride (salt) contained in all these waters will choke the life out of anyone attempting to drink them.

Throughout the ages, shipwrecked sailors and others have perished when their fresh water supply was exhausted. They tried to assuage their thirst with sea water, they lost their sense of reason through their intense thirst and drinking sea water resulted in their death.

Ocean water and other saline waters can be distilled.

Ocean water and salt lake waters can be distilled and pure sweet water obtained thereby. The sodium chloride and other mineral elements (except hydrogen and oxygen) will be left behind in the water container. The steam product is clear distilled water.

Sea Water is loaded with mineral elements.

Sea Water from the Oceans contains all the 16 gross mineral elements which are needed for the maintenance of the human body and, in addition, it contains all of the trace elements, 43 of them, of which the human body is composed. However, the sodium chloride is so highly concentrated that, in bulk, sea water is useless for human consumption.

Use only about 4 drops of Ocean
Water at a time. Just a squirt of it.

Sea water from the Oceans is of immense value when it is used in fractional amounts, at the rate of 4 to 8 drops of ocean water to the glass or pint of whatever beverage you plan to drink. We have used these drops of Ocean Water for a long time and we feel that we have derived much benefit from this practice. The Ocean Water we use is collected from the Pacific Coast of California and is called CATALINA SEA WATER. We get our supply in pint bottles from the Health Food Stores.

Ocean Water Is similar to human blood.

The analysis of Ocean Waters corresponds with a remarkable closeness to that of human blood. This fact has proved of great value in the needs for blood transfusions. At sea, when it is neither practical nor expedient to use human blood for transfusions, Ocean Waters have been used with great success and complete safety. As a matter of fact, sometimes Ocean Water has proved to be much safer than the use of human blood for transfusions.

Chapter 13

WATER IS WATER AND THAT'S THAT!

Oh, is that SO?

If you have NOT studied this book, or other books advocating the use of distilled water, DON'T discuss this subject with ANYONE! It is far better to let people THINK you know, than to expose yourself to the fact that the truth of the matter is not known to you, and that your opinion would be pure speculation.

There are differences in Water.

True, all water is liquid (above 32°F) and is wet, but to a degree the similarity between one water and another ends there.

Do you think Rain Water is pure?

There is rain water which, before it condenses from the clouds, is pure distilled water in vapor form. Once condensation sets in and water falls as rain then, on its way down to the earth, it becomes impregnated with whatever elements and pollution it can pick up from the atmosphere on its way down. Distilled water, even that which leaves the clouds, has the magnetic ability to collect whatever it contacts, if it is compatible with its absorption potential. Today, by the time rain water reaches the earth it is not much better than the Natural waters already here on earth.

Saline (salt) Waters:

There are Ocean and other saline waters which are not for drinking nor for food preparation purposes.

Consider Hard Water:

There is hard water which has very heavy calcium and magnesium and other mineral contents. When such hard water is steam distilled all the minerals and other substances are deposited in the bottom of the water container, while the steam travels towards its cooling channels to become pure distilled water.

Now consider Soft Water:
(Natural, or produced by Water Softeners).

Soft Water has its full complement of the minerals which it has picked up when in contact with soil and rocks. Calcium and magnesium are outstanding among these minerals. When soft water is used as a beverage or in the preparation of food, the mineral elements pass through the body and almost invariably leaves a residue of debris. Soft water can be easily distilled and thus becomes pure water without any mineral elements or other substances to worry about.

What value have Mineral Springs Waters?

There are innumerable Mineral Springs which contain an overabundance of one or more mineral elements. These waters have been used for ages in Health Spas and as Health Mineral Springs. These Spring Waters may undoubtedly have benefited some people, while the benefit to the majority may have been purely psychological. You know that the mind has a powerful influence on the body. If we think hard enough that a sulphur bath is what we need, we will soak ourselves in sulphur and go home feeling rewarded. To drink sulphur water is just as damaging in the long run as is any Natural water. However, even sulphur water can be distilled effectively.

To Drink — or NOT to Drink — Distilled Water?

Some people decry: DON'T drink Distilled Water! Other people say that if you drink any water, drink ONLY Distilled Water.

Who is right?

Consider the facts! The most conclusive argument will produce no more conviction to a closed mind than the most superficial assertion. There is no substitute for experience.

As I suggested in a preceding page, try the experiment of drinking ONLY Distilled Water, whenever you drink water, during the next 30 days, and drink at least 3 or 4 glasses of it a day. It may then dawn on you that there IS a vast difference between Distilled Water and Natural waters.

People who say DON'T drink Distilled Water because it leaches minerals out of your body, are 50% correct.

Those who recommend drinking ONLY Distilled Water are 100% correct.

What are the facts?

The sediment that cakes the bottom of the kettle in which Natural water has been boiled repeatedly, is clear visual evidence that steam has left the kettle, in the form of vapor-distilled water, while all the other contents of the water have cemented the bottom of the kettle.

These very same calcified elements which are left as residue in the kettle, and which are present in Natural waters, can be leached out of the body so long as they have not become a part of the cells and tissues of the body, if that were possible, which is unlikely.

Only the UNUSABLE minerals are leached out -
NOT those that are used in the tissues.

The minerals contained in Natural water are not of a kind which the cells of the body can use. Consequently they are rejected by the cells and constitute a hazard in the circulatory system. Distilled Water has the ability to collect these UN-usable minerals and pass them as sediment into the kidneys for excretion.

People who say that Distilled Water leaches minerals out of the body are, therefore, correct only in this respect. This is only 50% of the truth. It is virtually impossible for Distilled Water to separate minerals which have become an integral part of the cells and tissues of the body. Distilled water collects ONLY the minerals which remain in the body, minerals discarded from natural water AND from the cells, the minerals which the natural water originally collected from its contact with the earth and the rocks. Such minerals, having been rejected by the cells of the body are of no constructive value. On the contrary, they are debris which distilled water is capable of picking up and eliminating from the system.

Can Distilled Water separate
Caffeine from a cup of coffee? NO!

Distilled Water does not have the selective ability to separate detrimental substances which one has taken into the body by eating or drinking unwisely. If Distilled Water were able, for instance, to separate the caffeine from the numerous cups of coffee that a person drinks during a day, and pass it on directly to the kidneys for excretion, then such a person would not need to worry about the damage to his body which he is building up for a future affliction. As it is, millions of people drink coffee every day and these millions of people do not for a moment give any thought to the specter which awaits them in the form of disruption of the functions of the liver and kidneys and weakening the activity of the heart.

Atom by atom, calcium (lime) can become a 300 pound Mass.

I would remind you of the word picture in a preceding page about the 300 pounds of calcium or lime which, over the years, passes through the body of a person drinking Natural water. Such a load of lime anywhere, is not to be overlooked. Particularly when your own body is involved. If such a nightmare is not enough to make a person a devotee of Distilled Water, I would like to know what IS? It is not the glass of water you drink several times a day that is going to make you bedfast with calcified arteries in a week or two or a year or two. The effect is very slow, but nevertheless cumulative. It piles up a tiny bit at a time until it is too late to do anything about it. Prevention is the key note in the decision to use no water that is not Steam Distilled.

Warning - Ionized water is NOT Distilled Water!

There is a commercial product in the line of bottled water that features IONIZED (or DE-IONIZED) water. This is a process which is much too complicated to explain in a book of this type. There are some authorities that claim that the resin beds used as a base through which the water passes can become the breeding ground for bacteria, viruses, etc. Even though it is claimed that the process removes "practically" all of the mineral elements, and that it can be used for all "distilled water purposes", we prefer to use ONLY STEAM DISTILLED WATER.

To sum up the various kinds of water, there are Natural (or raw) water, hard water, soft water, boiled water, rain water (snow water is virtually rain water), filtered water, DISTAL (ionized or de-ionized) water and, finally, the "perfect" water: DISTILLED WATER.

We much prefer to be on the safe side and therefore use ONLY the PURE STEAM DISTILLED WATER.

Chapter 14
WATER IN MAN AND IN NATURE

Man can live without air for a matter of minutes, not much more. Man can live without water for only 3 or 4 days, although under certain circumstances and conditions he can survive for a week or two.

Men have died in 2 or 3 days in the desert, when unable to get a drop of water to drink, where even the night atmosphere is usually deficient of moisture. One man has been recorded as having died in 18 days by not drinking nor eating.

What is water doing In your body?.

The human body is composed of between 70 and 80 percent water. This is pure distilled water. It contains only those elements which it transports as inherent parts of the system, or such debris as is to be expelled from the body through the eliminative organs.

Cereals, bread, etc., do dehydrate one so much!

The most dehydrated people on earth are those who live on massive quantities of processed cereals, bread and meat, drinking very little water except perhaps in their coffee or tea and in soft drinks.

Processed cereals contain only from 7 to 13 percent water. The average water content of bread is only between 35 and 40 percent.

All plants contain distilled water.

Did you ever consider the amount of water needed to grow vegetation? Go into the country and look around. Notice that virtually everything on earth has water in its constitution. Every blade of grass, every bush, every plant, every tree is composed of 50 to 95 percent water. This is DISTILLED water, atmospheric and other water which the plant naturally and automatically distills. Roots raise the shoots out of the ground into the atmosphere and immediately the plant begins to collect and distill water from the atmosphere.

Without water this planet earth would perish!

Look up - and you will find the sky full of moisture, even though you cannot detect it as water. The invisible moisture is the distillation of the evaporation of the exposed surfaces of water in the oceans, lakes, rivers, etc. DISTILLED WATER is truly the life-blood of our planet earth.

Every ounce of fiber in vegetation needs
15 gallons in order to grow!

Vegetation constitutes the largest volume of products on earth, for our economy.

In their natural raw state, vegetables and fruits, nuts and seeds for man, grains and hay for animals, are composed of from 60 to 95 percent water. This is pure DISTILLED WATER.

This vegetation needs an average of 15 gallons of water for every single ounce of fiber in the plant while the plant is growing.

Believe it or not - It takes 20,000 gallons
of water to grow 100 lbs!

Just think! Nature supplies between 19,000 and 20,000 gallons of moisture and water in order to furnish man with every 100 pounds of vegetables and fruits, and with every 100 pounds of alfalfa and other feed for animals!

Get rid of One Gallon of water from your body every day!

The human body should expel about one gallon of moisture or liquid every 24 hours through the pores of the skin and through the other eliminative organs, to prevent the collection of excessive waste matter in the system. Without replenishment, the body would soon become dehydrated, besides becoming liable to debilitating ailments.

One rarely considers the amount of water which is obtained by means of the food one eats and the beverages one drinks during every 24 hours of one's life. This water problem should receive daily consideration and enough liquids should be used every day to replenish the water level of the body.

Don't fear decrepit old age - drink lots of Vegetable Juices.

All vegetables and fruits are replete with organic distilled water and their juices are the most nourishing. They are quickly assimilated in a fraction of the time necessary to digest and assimilate the vegetables and fruits themselves, as well as other foods. It is really essential, both for the well-being of the body and with the aim to avoid the long range likelihood of premature bodily decay, that at least a pint or two of Steam Distilled Water be drunk daily, plus as much fresh raw vegetable juices as possible.

Your own body creates some water within you!

We must, indeed, be grateful to our Creator for the wonderful, miraculous anatomy we have.

Just think how assiduously your body works for you to help prevent your destroying it, without your being the least bit conscious of the fact.

Consider the amazing manner in which, by its own inherent ability, the body is able to create a certain amount of its own distilled water by the oxidation of sugars, fats and proteins stored within it. The oxidation of one ounce of fat in the body, for instance, will produce one ounce of water!

Did you know that you are a human capsule filled 70% with water?

The purpose of drinking water is not solely for the quenching of thirst. Water constitutes the major part of the composition of the human body. More than 70% of the composition of the body is distilled water, whereas the body contains only about 5 quarts of blood!

The water in the human system must essentially be distilled water because distilled water, by its inherent magnetic principle, is able to collect many of the impurities which either collect in mass or float around in the system.

Hot or cold - the water within you keeps you temperate.

The water in the body is necessary to maintain the body at the temperature best suited to its comfort in accord with its environment. This is accomplished by means of the temperature control mechanism in the brain area, by a group of fibers known as the Hypothalamus. We will discuss this gland-like organism in due course.

What would a woman do without water to pour out in tears?

Water is needed in your breathing processes. You know how uncomfortable it is to have your nostrils so dry that they irritate, while, on the other hand, your nostrils are equally bothersome when they become overly moist with excessive fluids. In more or less the same area, a deficiency of water in the lachrymal glands would make it virtually impossible for a woman to weep when under emotional stress, and that of course would be calamitous under many circumstances!

When water supply fails, eat lots of vegetables and fruits.

As the need to supply the body with so much water is obvious, the source of the water is an important matter. Distilled Water, we have emphasized, is truly of vital importance. In the fresh raw vegetable and fruit juices we obtain not only the finest distilled water available, but also the nourishment which will thoroughly and speedily feed the cells of the body most successfully. Such a constructive and preventive program cannot help but develop Vibrant Health and forestall the nightmare of waning energy and vitality.

Through lack of this vital knowledge, people take water for granted when they are thirsty or when they are preparing food. Water is such a common commodity that rarely does anyone give it a second thought, so long as it is available. When water becomes scarce or is lacking altogether, whether by accident or through Natural causes, few people realize how much water is available that lies hidden within vegetables and fruits, even eaten whole, in their natural raw state.

Water supplies you with heat and energy.

You need distilled water in your system if you want heat and energy. The food you eat does more for you than to nourish the cells of your body. It furnishes you with heat and energy, if the food is the kind and type of nourishment that will supply you with these commodities. Bear in mind that 25 per cent of the heat value of the food you eat is dissipated by perspiration through the pores of your skin as well as through your lungs when you breathe. This evaporation alone expels between one and two pints of water from your system every day.

The loss of water through the pores of your skin becomes more pronounced in hot weather, and particularly when strenuous exercise is indulged in, when perspiration increases greatly. In the case of such copious perspiration the body can readily lose ONE GALLON of water in one hour's time.

How do you lose water in your system?

Besides the loss of water by perspiration, between the elimination of liquids by the kidneys and the excreta from the bowels there can be an average loss of some 2 to 3 quarts of water in the course of 24 hours.

With an excessive consumption of beverages this elimination is correspondingly increased. This is particularly the case when beer is consumed in too great quantities, as we have told you in detail in a preceding page.

Chapter 15

THE SALIVARY GLANDS

Those glands in your mouth. They need water constantly

Among the many functions of the body using water constantly, we must not overlook the salivary glands. Without the salivary glands you would not be able to digest your food and your mouth would be perpetually dry enough to drive you out of your mind!

There are three types of salivary glands, and you should become acquainted with them because they will intensify your interest in maintaining the proper water balance in your system.

The parotid glands are located one in each cheek. The submandibular glands (mandible means jaw) are in the rear of your mouth under your jaw. The sublingual glands (lingua is the tongue) are located under your tongue. *Study the accompanying sketch.*

Besides the salivary glands, the tongue itself has a number of glands with pores opening on its surface. These are the serous glands (serous means thin or watery), and the mucous glands on the upper side of the tongue, and mixed glands on the under-surface.

The salivary glands are specifically active in the digestive processing of the food and beverages which you put in your mouth. The tongue glands, on the other hand, are constantly active in keeping the mouth and the tongue moist.

The combined liquid output of these glands amounts to about 3 pints every 24 hours. Realize how important it is to use PURE water!

Can you imagine what an accumulation of calcium (lime) would taste like in your mouth if the unusable minerals are not completely eliminated from your body?

Where do these glands get their constant water supply?

Yes, where do these glands get their moisture? From the distilled water which is constantly circulating through your system. From the water storage in your body!

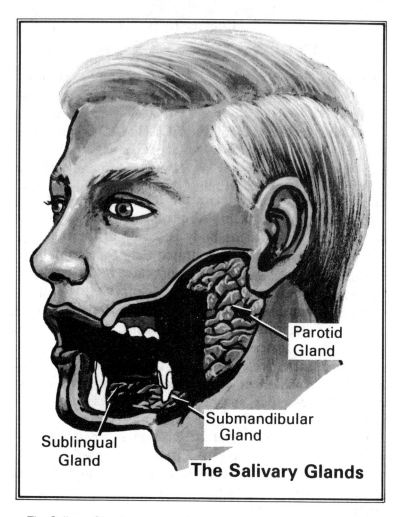

Parotid Gland

Submandibular Gland

Sublingual Gland

The Salivary Glands

The Salivary Glands secrete saliva to start the digestive process. There are other glands, on the top and on the under side of the tongue whose function is to keep the tongue and the mouth moist, constantly. (As the tongue is not shown on this sketch, these particular moisture-producing glands cannot be shown.)

All these glands use about 3 pints of water a day. If such water is deficient or in any way polluted, dryness of the tongue and mouth can ensue. The tongue and mouth would then be uncomfortably dry, and the saliva would be inadequate or deficient enough to prevent the proper initial steps of digestion. This could result in heart burn, indigestion, etc.

The careful selection of all beverages is obviously of the greatest importance.

Chapter 16

WATER STORAGE IN YOUR BODY

Water in Your Muscles!

The storage of water in the body brings to light a very interesting problem. Approximately 15 to 16 percent of the water in your body is stored in your muscles. When muscles become dehydrated they become flabby.

When there is a deficiency of water in the muscles, and when the circulating water happens to leave a residue of unusable minerals in the muscles, very painful muscular affliction can result during physical exercise. Exercise causes the muscles to expand and contract and when there is dehydration, and in the presence of extraneous substances, (such as calcium and magnesium residues), muscular spasms, cramps, anguish, agony, torment and torture make the victim very miserable.

Meat creates Uric Acid in the Body!

There is another enemy of muscular comfort which thrusts its painful darts into muscular regions. It is uric acid.

Where does uric acid come from? It is the end product of the excessive eating of meat and meat products. Digestion of meat causes the generation of uric acid. Muscles have a particular affinity for uric acid - up to a certain point. Muscles have a limit of tolerance for uric acid which they can absorb with impunity. When the limit of tolerance has been reached and exceeded, uric acid forms very fine sharp crystals which pierce the nerves in order, perhaps, to warn the victim that he is guilty of having become a carnivorous person. These sharp uric acid crystals are nothing to be treated lightly nor to be neglected. When neglected, the victim is punished by afflictions such as rheumatism, neuritis, and the like.

People who eat no meat are rarely troubled with these uric acid afflictions. Such vegetarians, however, are never exempt from nor immune to the afflictions resulting from the accumulation of calcium and magnesium residues collected over the years in their veins and arteries. The deposits of these elements left there by the Natural waters used as beverages and for food preparation, if not corrected, will leave their mark in later years, also causing muscle trouble.

The skin is also a reservoir.

Water is also stored in the skin in amounts ranging from 10 to 15 percent. In order to keep the skin in prime condition it is necessary to maintain a correct balance of water and fats. The deficiency or the poor quality of the water used as a beverage has a profound bearing on the quality of the skin.

Drinking a sufficient amount of distilled water daily can be a great help to keep the skin clear, and drinking vegetable juices furnish the finest nourishment we have found for maintaining the texture of beautiful skin.

Chapter 17
ABOUT CARROT JUICE

Carrot Juice - truly a boon to humanity, when health is wanted.
For more than half a century I have been using quantities of carrot juice daily, anywhere from a pint to, at times, a gallon a day. I attribute my Vibrant Health and the splendid texture of my skin directly to the use of carrot juice.

Utterly ignore those who know not what they talk about!
There was a time, when I first started drinking carrot juice, that my skin took on an orange yellow hue. I discovered that this was due to the cleansing of my liver, which happened to be in VERY bad condition at the time. However, after a few months the discoloration disappeared and my skin was better and clearer than it had ever been.

During the past half century, thousands upon thousands, if not MILLIONS of people have been drinking carrot juice with NEVER, to my knowledge, a single adverse effect.

Newspapers are notorious for stacks of misinformation!
I am emphasizing this here now, because some columnists have taken it upon themselves to challenge the beneficial use of carrot juice and to attack the benefits which millions of people the world over have received from its use. This silly twaddle causes confusion in the mind of some who earnestly seek to improve their health and their lot in life. It is unnecessary. Anyone challenging the value of fresh raw vegetable juices as a means to gain or regain health, energy and vitality has certainly had no experience. As there is no substitute for experience, it would be far better if they tried a 6 month's raw vegetable juice regimen.

RAW CARROT JUICE
Depending on the condition of the individual, raw carrot juice may be taken indefinitely in any reasonable quantities—from one to six or eight pints a day. It has the effect of helping to normalize the entire system. It is the richest source of Vitamin A which the body can quickly assimilate and contains also an ample supply of Vitamins B, C, D, E, G, and K. It helps to promote the appetite and is an aid to digestion.

It is a valuable aid in the improvement and maintenance of the bone structure of the teeth.

Raw carrot juice is a natural solvent for ulcerous and cancerous conditions. It is a resistant to infections, doing most efficient work in conjunction with the adrenal glands. It helps prevent infections of the eyes and throat as well as the tonsils and sinuses and the respiratory organs generally. It also protects the nervous system and is unequalled for increasing vigor and vitality.

Intestinal and liver diseases are sometimes due to a lack of certain of the elements contained in properly prepared raw carrot juice. When this is the case, then a noticeable cleaning up of the liver may take place, and the material which was clogging it may be found to dissolve. Frequently this is released so abundantly that the intestinal and urinary channels are inadequate to care for this overflow, and in a perfectly natural manner it is passed into the lymph for elimination from the body by means of the pores of the skin. This material has a distinctly orange or yellow pigment and while it is being so eliminated from the body will sometimes discolor the skin. Whenever such a discoloration takes place after drinking carrot or other juices, it is an indication that the liver is getting a well-needed cleansing.

The endocrine glands, especially the adrenals and the gonads, require food elements found in raw carrot juice. Sterility is sometimes overcome by its use. The cause of sterility has been traced to the continuous use of foods in which atoms and enzymes were destroyed by cooking or pasteurizing.

Dry skin, dermatitis, and other skin blemishes are due to a deficiency in the body of some of these food elements contained in carrot juice. This is also a factor in eye trouble, as in ophthalmia, conjunctivitis, etc.

As an aid to dissolve ulcers and cancer, raw carrot juice has proved itself the miracle of the age. It was found essential, however, that it be properly prepared and every vestige of concentrated sugar, starch and flour of every kind be completely eliminated from the diet.

Carrot juice is composed of a combination of elements which nourish the entire system, helping to normalize its weight as well as its chemical balance.

Due to the deficiency of live atoms in the food people have been eating, particularly during the present and immediately preceding generations, the starved and half-starved body cells, unable to function properly and efficiently the way they are intended to, rebel and become disorganized. Not being entirely dead these cells become dislodged from their anchorage (figuratively speaking), and float around until they find some location within the human anatomy where they can group together. With the entire body suffering more or less from live atoms starvation, there are plenty of locations in the body where protective resistance is low.

We must not conclude that ulcers and cancer result only from physical imperfections. As we have already pointed out, these ailments and many others may very likely stem from lifelong resentments, from stress due to states of mind such as jealousy, fear, hate, worry, frustration, and other negative intangible impediments. These are the first things to be dissolved and banished. Nevertheless we must not overlook the fact that Malnutrition and failure to maintain the system in the highest possible state of cleanliness within and without, and mentally, may definitely also be contributing factors.

My book, FRESH VEGETABLE AND FRUIT JUICES, What's Missing In Your Body? is based on my experience over many score years, and is attested to by innumerable people the world over.

Chapter 18
THE DEADLY CHLORINE

The present-day history books give little if any details about the chlorine gas that was so despicably used during World War One. Untold thousands of soldiers and civilians outlived the end of the war as wrecks, with their inward parts burned by chlorine gas.

Chlorine kills the enemy in war and the Citizens in peace!

When the war was over, the use of chlorine was diverted to poison germs in our drinking water. The idea was conceived, and carried out, to chlorinate ALL water supplies throughout the country with the avowed object of killing bacteria.

Chlorine + animal fats = Atherosclerosis

The combination of Chlorine (when used in chlorinated water) combined with animal fats eaten in the diet, causes a chemical amalgamation of the chlorine and the fat which results in the formation of a gummy substance in the arteries. This gummy substance is a cumulative process so long as the person continues to drink and eat this combination. There is no way to correct this affliction once it has progressed too far, because the accumulated gummy product in the arteries causes heart attacks as the mildest warning, likely to develop into atherosclerosis, then a funeral.

What is the answer?

The answer is simple. When steam leaves the container in which the water has been boiled to convert it into DISTILLED WATER, neither the chlorine, the minerals nor the toxins and poisons join the DISTILLED WATER!

Chapter 19

CONNECTIVE TISSUES

These are membranes covering and supporting everything in the body.

When a large volume of Natural water is consumed, osmotic pressure (which is the pressure produced by osmosis) is demonstrably decreased, causing the obstruction of functions and activities in whatever area it may affect. This interference with the osmotic pressure may result from the mineral matter in the water or from an excessive consumption of salt and starchy and sugary foods.

The connective tissues are films of varying fineness, forming a membrane the vast extent of which is beyond the conception of the human mind. While I have no actual figures upon which to base an estimate, it seems to me that if all the connective tissues in the body were separated and stretched out on the ground, they would cover several ACRES!

My Friends' Station Wagon had a head attack!

Early this year a gentleman and his wife, friends of ours, decided to go away for a few days. Their itinerary to the Northern end of Arizona took them through the town of Williams (6800 feet elevation above sea level) to the City of Flagstaff (6905 feet elevation), a distance of some 50 miles. Half way to Flagstaff they drove into a heavy snow storm. The wife was driving, when they were about half way to Flagstaff the engine in their station wagon began to have heart trouble. That's right. Their ENGINE had heart trouble!

He told his wife to pull over to the side of the road a 4-lane highway and he drove the car at about 15 miles an hour (as against the 50 miles an hour she was driving), nursing it along until they arrived safely in Flagstaff where he drove directly into the Service Station of the Dealer who handled the same kind of car as theirs.

He told the foreman he thought the gasoline line from the gas tank to the carburetor might be clogged up.

The foreman quickly took the filter off the gas line and replaced it with a clean new one, whereupon the engine purred like a kitten and they went on their way. He tells me they have had no further trouble. The diagnosis was correct!

The filter on my friends' gas line is analogous to ONE tiny particle of connective tissue. They bought a new filter and had it connected, in a matter of minutes. If you should have a heart attack you cannot replace the connective tissue, at any price. The harm has been done, irretrievably. The accumulation of lime (calcium) and magnesium, over a period of 40 or 50 years of drinking Natural Waters can readily be quite considerable. Such an accumulation of calcium could block many filtering places in the connective tissues, besides veins and arteries.

Connective tissues are the greatest filtering plant in the world!

Every drop of water, lymph and blood which circulates through the body is filtered through these connective tissues. Consequently all the food you eat, after it is digested, is likewise filtered through these connective tissues before its component particles can reach the cells for which they are intended. When, through such filtering, the connective tissues are blocked with either calcium, white flour starch and other incompatible substances, then the blocked areas are bound to cause trouble.

Oh how refined foods do impede the filtering processes!

The impurities which circulate through the system with the water and the blood are the villains which clog up the microscopically fine mesh of the filtering membrane. Such foods as concentrated devitalized flour, starches and sugars, in addition to the calcium in the water, can do their share in obstructing the passages through the connective tissues.

It is important to bear this in mind because we cannot blame only the calcium, magnesium, etc., in the water for these obstructions. Wrong food combinations as well as starch and sugar products in the carbohydrate category can be the culprits. There are the right and nourishing kind of carbohydrates, and there are the wrong kind intended to appease the appetite without regard to either their health or their nourishing qualities.

What Carbohydrates are nourishing, compatible foods?

The carbohydrates which are considered nourishing foods are vegetables and fruits, potatoes, beans, lentils, herbs, peas, grains, etc., when eaten raw and, in the case of beans, peas and lentils, and grains, when sprouted.

The carbohydrates that are in "refined" foods have been deprived of their nourishing value, and we do not consider them compatible with the achievement of Vibrant Health.

What's wrong with "refining" foods?

The refining processes consist of REMOVING the valuable part of the food. In other words whatever will prevent the food from being kept for long periods of time without spoiling, is extracted and eliminated. These "refined" products are the carbohydrates which are not soluble in water and can therefore readily block the connective tissues, particularly the veins and arteries. Examples of this effect are noticeable in choked varicose veins, coronary occlusions causing heart attacks, etc.

What Is the purpose of Connective Tissues?

In general, the purpose of connective tissues is to bind, to support and to protect the parts and organs in which they are involved. These parts include the millions of walls of blood vessels, the miles of nerves and nerve sheathing, the muscles, the glands, etc. Their inherent function is in connection with the circulation and storage of body fluids and of nutritional substances.

The connective tissues consist of membranes forming adipose tissues, pigment tissues, the walls of the blood vessels, the membranes supporting organs such as the liver, the kidneys, the testicles, etc. They are also involved in the metabolism of cells.

Some of the connective tissues have cells for the collection of fats. When these "fat-cells" become engorged with fatty substances they form the membrane known as adipose tissue.

Connective tissues form the structure of the cornea of the eyes, the outer covering of the brain, and the membrane of the spinal cord.

Every piece and parcel of connective tissues is intimately involved in the filtering of water. THAT is why the kind and the quality of the water is so important. Obviously no better nor safer water can be used than Distilled Water. This is the reason for my detailed and lengthy dissertation on the subject of connective tissues.

I assume you value YOUR health, and furthermore you surely do not want to join the throng of prematurely aged people who have nothing to look forward to but for a demise.

You can't tell where or when calcium
WILL obstruct the filters!

So vast is the area of the connective tissues that it would be quite impossible to guess where a filtering process will be blocked. The most frequent location is of course in the veins and arteries because the fluids circulate through every part of these channels constantly and take the brunt of the traffic.

Remember, that while you have only about 5 quarts of blood in your body, you have between 50 and 80 quarts of water throughout your system. Watch the water you put into your system, if you value VIBRANT HEALTH.

Chapter 20

YOUR GLANDS NEED DISTILLED WATER

Are you acquainted with your Endocrine Glands?

I can state without fear of contradiction that your Endocrine Glands, your Glands of Internal Secretion, are by far the most important and vital organs in your body.

Even without much knowledge of your anatomy, you could profitably spend hours on end studying the Endocrine Gland Chart which I composed and drew for the benefit of anybody concerned, and interested.

In my opinion you could study any one of the books I have in my library on the subject of these Glands, 400 and 500 page books, and not get so clear a picture in a matter of days, as you should in the pictorial study of my Endocrine Gland Chart, in a matter of minutes.

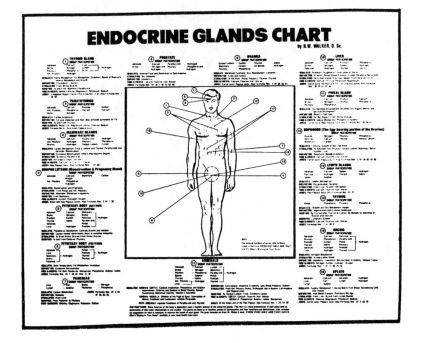

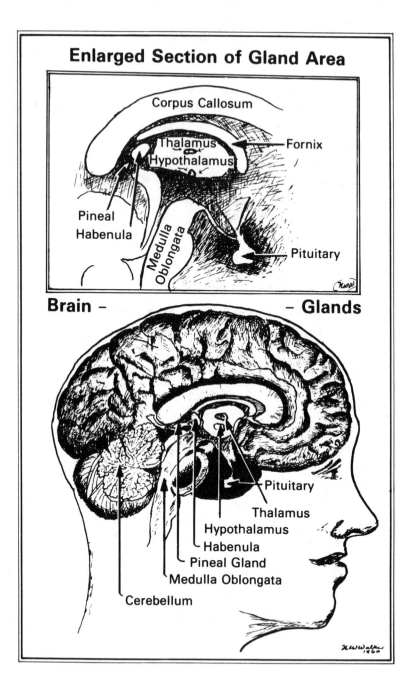

Enlarged Section of Gland Area

Corpus Callosum

Thalamus

Hypothalamus

Fornix

Pineal

Habenula

Medulla Oblongata

Pituitary

Brain –   – Glands

Pituitary

Thalamus

Hypothalamus

Habenula

Pineal Gland

Medulla Oblongata

Cerebellum

Chapter 21

THE HYPOTHALAMUS

The Hypothalamus is a glandular organ. It is composed of a group of fibers and is located in the midsection of the brain. Although the hypothalamus is not an Endocrine Gland, it could be considered the Emperor of the Endocrine Glands system.

(Note: Because the Hypothalamus is not actually an Endocrine Gland, it is not shown on my Endocrine Gland Chart).

Located just above the pituitary gland and just below the thalamus, it is involved in, regulates, controls, stimulates and inhibits one or other of all the glands in the body, thus having a direct influence over virtually every activity of the human system. Study the accompanying illustrations.

Water balance is extremely important.

The control of the water in the system is both important and far reaching, because it is essential to maintain the body fluid in balance, which means regulating the conservation of the fluid, the replenishment and the elimination of water.

It is one of the functions of the hypothalamus to take care of these activities for you. Naturally, the best water available is none too good for your system and for the activity of your glands. Distilled Water is one answer to this problem which may make the difference between a healthy system or an ailing body.

Elimination of water from body must be under control.

Without regulated control, the urinary bladder would let so much liquid escape that a human being could not function normally and would, furthermore, become dehydrated in a very short time.

The hypothalamus exerts this control, through the pituitary gland. In doing so, the quality of the water in the system has a marked influence, and this is something that is never considered when one is thirsty.

Did you ever feel too hot or too cold?

In the Winter time, one shivers when it is cold. In the Summer one perspires when the heat becomes intense and humid. What is the answer? *Temperature regulation!*

In the home, office and factory we have thermostats which automatically control the necessary temperature. In your body you have the hypothalamus which is your temperature regulating mechanism.

In cold weather the nerve impulses act in closing many of the pores of the skin and at the same time raising the heat factor in the blood circulation. This causes the individual to generate his own furnace heat, so to speak.

In hot weather, on the other hand, another set of impulses is started which opens up the pores and permits moisture to wet the skin, resulting in the cool feeling of air against the moist skin, and to bring a cool degree of comfort to the system.

These impulses involve the action of nerves, and nerves have a constant flow of cerebrospinal fluid through them which is dependent on the quality of the fluid in the body.

Hungry? Your Hypothalamus tells you so!

Hunger and appetite are of course two totally different sensations, but they are both under the direction of the hypothalamus.

When the cells and tissues of your body have been active, they need replenishment and regeneration. This is taken care of by the hypothalamus sending the necessary impulses to the digestive organs and glands. This is hunger.

Appetite, however, rings another bell. In this case it is the desire elements in the brain areas that nudge the hypothalamus into the suggestive activity to eat or drink what the brain has indicated.

Obesity is rarely the result of hunger but it is definitely associated with the hypothalamus responding to the appetite desires. Thus we understand why appetite is or can be under the control of the will and will power.

Your blood pressure responds to orders from the Hypothalamus!

The needs of the body for the flow and pressure of the blood varies constantly. The regulation of blood pressure involves not only the action of the heart, but also is initiated by the hypothalamus.

If you had studied anatomy in your school days, you would know that the dilation (the enlarging or expanding) and the constriction of your blood vessels is an essential process in maintaining the proper pressure balance of blood in your system.

The volume and the quality of the water in your blood has a great influence in the state of your health. The adrenal glands exert much

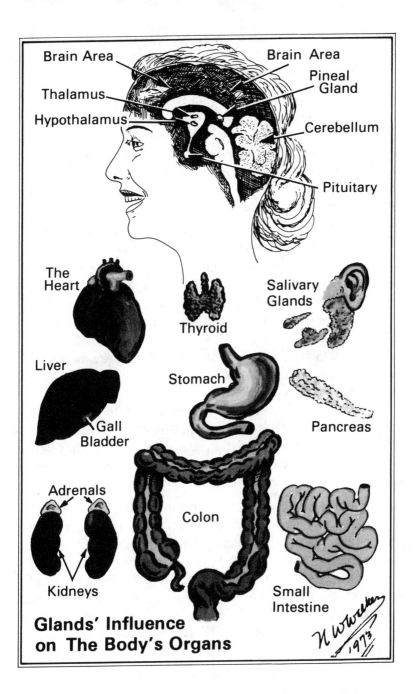

**Glands' Influence
on The Body's Organs**

69

of the control of these processes, but the adrenal glands are themselves influenced by the hypothalamus. Thus the quality of the water in the system affects your entire glandular chain.

Calcium (lime) from regular water may play havoc with the Glands.

Distilled water is always the safest to drink. As regular water may leave deposits of calcium and other unwanted minerals in the blood circulation, these may find their way into the Endocrine Glands system with disastrous results which might never be attributed to these unusable minerals as the cause.

If one in a million is afflicted by such lime deposits, Don't You be the One!

Because billions upon billions of people in the past several thousand years have survived the drinking of regular water, the real cause of their demise was never attributed to calcium deposits in their system. Today we have every reason to suppose than such has been the case.

However, there is no cause for alarm. People are indoctrinated with the idea that man's life span is a mere 3 score and 10, so (they think) Why worry about it?

Personally, I will not go on that premise, of Why worry about it? I prefer to "play it safe", so that my liquid beverage intake is and in so far as I can control it, will be till the end of my days, fresh raw vegetable and fruit juices (which ARE distilled water) and as much distilled water every day as I feel the need of.

Hypothalamus Involved in all your body and mental activities.

In my search to find the involvement of the hypothalamus in all the physical and mental activities of the body and of the individual as a personality, I have failed to find a single instance in which the hypothalamus does not have a direct or indirect influence. Therefore the intelligent conclusion is, that nutrition in liquid and substance is of vital importance to health, energy, vigor, vitality and longevity, and should therefore be chosen and used as intended by Nature.

Study the picture "Glands' Influence on the body's Organs" herein.

Can sleep - or cannot sleep?

When you're lying awake with a dismal headache and repose is taboo'd by anxiety, sit up in bed for a moment and realize that there is something or other disturbing your hypothalamus. That's right. That is the mechanism that controls your going to sleep and your waking up.

Do you ever get angry, resentful, exasperated, bitter, furious?

While your Solar Plexus, in your midriff, is considered the seat of the emotions, your adrenal glands and your thyroid gland are just as deeply involved. Nevertheless, the very seat of emotional involvement is your hypothalamus. Think of this when your emotions have the tendency to get the better of you. As you learn to control your hypothalamus, not only by means of the right food you eat and the constructive beverages you drink, but also by the use of your mind and will power, all your glands will benefit and cooperate with your attaining peace and tranquillity within you.

Chapter 22
THE PITUITARY

The pituitary is the gland immediately below the hypothalamus. It generates a hormone which is involved in the movement of water throughout the body. It is known as an antidiuretic hormone whose vital function is so important that a deficiency of this hormone or its absence will cause the disturbing ailment known as diabetes insipidus.

Osmosis transfers liquids and the substances they contain from the veins and arteries through the microscopic capillary veins inside the walls of the blood vessels to be distributed to the places they are intended for. To define, osmosis is the passage of liquids, concentrated solutions and vapors through semipermeable membranes or skin. The fluidity of water in the blood and lymphatic streams is dependent on the correct balance of water in both. Any blockage or interference with the freedom of this flow results in the occlusion, if not the actual closure of blood vessels. This may even be fatal.

Billions of people have died from drinking regular water, died prematurely, without anybody even realizing that the lime in the water was the culprit.

However, billions of people are drinking regular natural waters today, and are alive and apparently healthy, so - why worry? If you don't care about your own future? It's Your body, anyway, and it's Your life. Just go ahead and do what you want with it.

The Pituitary cannot select the
kind of water. That is up to You!

The pituitary gland works in a more or less automatic manner and only within the scope of its own functions. It is not able to distinguish between polluted and distilled water.

When an individual drinks a large quantity of liquids, more than is his custom, nerve impulses are projected from the hypothalamus to the pituitary to urgently take care of this abnormal volume of liquids. If the liquids are free of interfering substances and minerals, the hormones activating the kidneys will function normally.

If the beverages are incompatible or inconsistent with the normal functioning of these hormones and with the processes of fluid elimination, then the condition develops known as diuresis, or an abnormal flow of urine. Obstructions in the form of kidney stones develop all too often when one consumes beverages containing such minerals as calcium and magnesium. Distilled water could avoid this hazard.

The Pituitary has a vast and varied mission to perform!

The functions of the pituitary are as vast as they are varied, but they are concentrated mainly in connection with directing the blood supply (which includes also its lymph and water content) to the heart, to the liver, to the thyroid gland, to the pancreas, to the adrenal glands, to the bones and to the reproductive glands, the ovaries and the testes.

Bear in mind that your body contains only about 5 quarts of blood, while the water present in the constitution of your body is equivalent to about 70% of the weight of your body. In other words, if you weigh about 150 pounds, your body would contain about 80 quarts or about 20 gallons of water in the constitution of your anatomy. If these estimates are correct, then every man and woman who died before reaching the age of 120 years during the past 4,200 years may possibly have perished by reason of occlusion of the blood vessels caused by the unusable minerals in the water which they drank throughout their lives.

This hypothesis is understandable when you realize that the water in your system circulates through every part of your body with the blood and the lymph, constantly bathing every cell and tissue in your anatomy. Naturally, if the water you drink is pure distilled water, it will be free from all extraneous substances and there would be no danger of occlusions from this source.

Chapter 23

THE THYROID GLAND

Has a direct relation to the Pituitary.

The functions of the thyroid are controlled by the pituitary "thyrotropic" hormone which releases and controls the production of the thyroid hormone thyroxin The thyroid is one of the two most vascular glands in the system. By vascular we mean replete with ducts or vessels conveying water, blood and lymph. This is a very important situation when you realize that every drop of blood, with its water and lymph contents, passes through the thyroid every 15 minutes throughout your life. If any impurities are deposited in the thyroid during the time the blood is passing through it, it is likely to cause the gland to enlarge. This condition is commonly referred to as "goiter".

The Thyroid makes giants and dwarfs.

An exophthalmic goiter is a toxic goiter. The result of which is an overly active thyroid that causes weight loss, nervousness, and protruding eyeballs in both children and adults. Cretinism is the result of an under active thyroid. It is a word that describes the physical malformation, and the arrested mental and sexual development that is caused in children who suffer from a deficiency of thyroid secretion.

In adults, an under-active thyroid results in great mental and physical loss of vigor, often increase in weight and loss of hair.

The nerve supply to the thyroid is derived from the brain area, a delicate situation when the water and blood carry too many impurities and leave too many of them deposited in the vascular system of the thyroid. Just look at the picture of the Thyroid!

It seems as if everything points to the use of Distilled Water.

With all the 5 quarts of blood, and no telling how much of the water in your system passing through your thyroid about 100 times every 24 hours, it is certainly worth giving a second thought before eating and drinking anything that may affect the body adversely. It really pays to be alert.

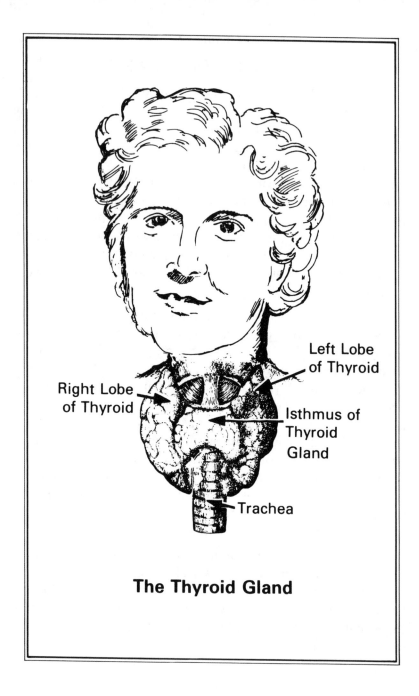

Left Lobe of Thyroid

Right Lobe of Thyroid

Isthmus of Thyroid Gland

Trachea

The Thyroid Gland

Chapter 24

THE ADRENAL GLANDS

In ancient Bible days these were referred to as the "reins'.

The adrenal glands, two capsules located on the top of each of the two kidneys, are probably the most prolific hormone manufacturers in the entire human system. They secrete or generate about 48 hormones of diverse kinds and types.

So far-reaching are their functions and activities that it is little wonder that the "reins" are referred to more than 15 times throughout the Holy Bible.

No chain is stronger than its weakest link.

The efficiency of the functions of the adrenal hormones, no less than the efficiency of the functions of the entire chain of Endocrine Glands, can, like a chain, be no stronger than its weakest link.

We look for that link in both the blood and the water supply. The blood carries the appropriate nourishment to the thyroid, as it does to every other part of the body, and the water comes along to wash out impurities. But the water must itself be pure if it is to do its task efficiently.

The adrenal glands are essential for the preservation of life as well as for life activities. When there is a deficiency in the requirements of these glands the fluid balance of the body is correspondingly disrupted, *which could prevent your feeling pain when you may need a "pain-alert".*

Pain is not an ailment in any sense of the word. It is the alert, the warning, that there is something amiss in your system.

It is essential that we feel pain, shock, cold, unpredictable muscular over-exertion, emotional agitation. These are all warnings that unless we do something to correct what has gone amiss, something worse will befall us.

The adrenal hormone adrenaline is secreted the instant heart trouble develops or the blood pressure does not behave itself.

Epinephrine is another adrenal hormone. It causes the liver to release sugar from its storage bins to raise the blood sugar level.

Study the accompanying sketch of the Adrenal Glands.

The Adrenal Glands regulate your metabolism.

Much of the digestion and assimilation of your food is regulated by the activity of the adrenal glands by their involvement in your metabolism.

Just as the activities of the adrenal glands are prolific, so are also the disturbances which can result from interference with their tasks. The disfunction of these glands can result in tumors, convulsions and even in trouble with the visual apparatus, particularly in connection with the retina of the eyes.

It certainly IS worthwhile to drink plenty of distilled water.

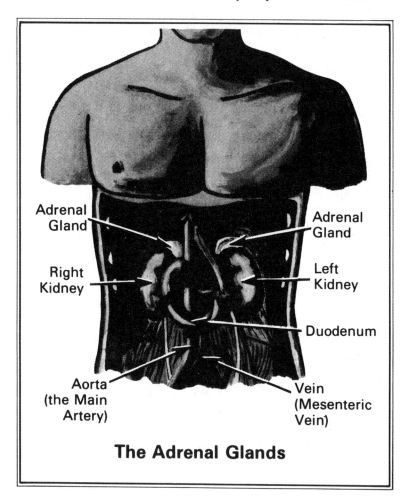

The Adrenal Glands

Chapter 25

THE PANCREAS

The Pancreas is a double gland. It has two functions.

The pancreas is a tremendously important gland in which the blood, the lymph and water play a vital part.

One part furnishes digestive juices.

The pancreatic duct runs the whole length of the pancreas and joins the bile duct, the channel through which bile flows into the duodenum from the gall bladder. Together, the bile and the pancreatic juice form an important digestive juice in which water forms an essential constituent.

Water is supplied to the pancreas with the circulation of the blood and lymph. Impurities in the water content affect the quality of the digestive juices, resulting in food being improperly digested.

Another part furnishes Insulin.

There is a part of the pancreas which contains about one million cells within a limited area which are known as the Islands of Langerhans. Like every other cell in the body, these cells are constantly bathed in liquid.

These cells are glands of internal secretion, which means that they generate a hormone, known as Insulin, which is injected directly into the blood. Insulin serves to regulate the metabolism of carbohydrates and the blood-sugar level.

A disturbance in the production of insulin results in what is known as diabetes mellitus. In this ailment the body is not able to use the blood sugar which increases in volume in the blood and has to be excreted through the kidneys. For this reason this type of diabetes is also known as sugar-diabetes.

The sometimes excessive use of starchy and sugar foods is the incipient cause of this disease, and it is aggravated when the water carries too great a load of unusable minerals. Distilled water is a safer water to drink, and the use of the proper fresh raw vegetable juices is of immense value in helping the pancreas to function efficiently.

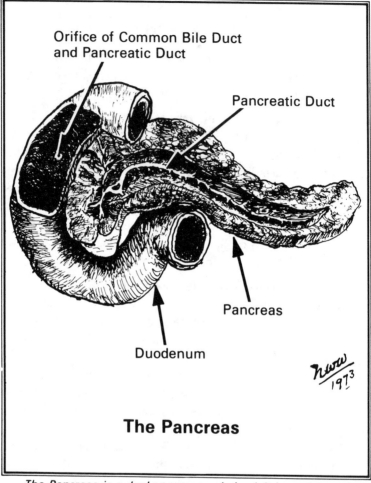

Orifice of Common Bile Duct
and Pancreatic Duct

Pancreatic Duct

Pancreas

Duodenum

The Pancreas

The Pancreas is a dual or compound gland. It is analogous in its structure to the salivary glands.

It generates the pancreatic digestive juices which flow into the duodenum from the pancreatic duct. It then combines with the bile from the gall bladder through the joint or common bile duct within the duodenum.

In the pancreas there is also a group of about a million cells known as the islands of langerhans. By means of internal secretion these generate the hormone insulin which is injected directly into the blood.

Chapter 26

THE LIVER

Everything you eat and drink passes through the liver.

The liver is the laboratory of the digestive system. Everything that has been processed by the small intestine which can pass through the walls of the intestine is picked up by the blood and the water which accompanies the blood, and taken directly into the liver.

In the liver, metabolism takes place. Fats are broken down to furnish heat and energy. Carbohydrates are disintegrated to form sugars, and proteins are broken down into their individual amino acids thus producing urea. Urea, when excessive, is collected in the muscles and forms into uric acid crystals. These crystals eventually are so sharp and numerous that they prick the nerve sheathe and you then know what rheumatism, neuritis, etc., feel like!

Vitamin "A" is a very important Vitamin, and it is stored in the liver. Carotene is the most prolific source of Vitamin "A" and carrot juice is the means by which we can obtain Vitamin "A" in abundance. As a matter of fact, sometimes when a large amount of carrot juice is consumed over an extended period of time, it may cause the skin to acquire temporarily a yellow or orange hue. This discoloration is not the carrot juice coming out of the skin. It is the stale bile from the liver and gall bladder which was not eliminated in the course of events in the past, and which the juice helps to eliminate through the kidneys, and through the skin.

The liver generates bile and it is stored in the gall bladder for use in the digestive processes. The combination of carrot-beet-and cucumber juice, in addition to the use of Distilled Water, has been found to be very helpful in cleansing the body of stale bile.

The skin is the most extensive eliminative organ in the body. When discoloration takes place after drinking much carrot juice, the color will eventually disappear, leaving a skin more beautiful than it was in the past.

Carrot Juice is one of the most healthy and complete foods which the human body can obtain. There is no deleterious effect from drinking quantities of carrot juice. I personally, have consumed ONE GALLON of carrot juice daily, when I felt the need with most beneficial results. To this very day I drink all the carrot juice (plus other vegetable juices) that I have the time and inclination to drink. Don't let anybody tell you that fresh raw carrot and other vegetable juices are anything BUT healthy and helpful. Read my book FRESH VEGETABLE AND FRUIT JUICES, What's Missing In Your Body? It is recognized the world over as the most helpful and authoritative book on this subject. Remember that ALL fresh raw vegetable, and fruit, juices consist of Distilled Water distilled by Nature!

As the liver is such a delicate and active gland, its supply of water and the quality of the water it receives is of vital concern to anyone who values Vibrant Health and longevity.

Chapter 27

THE KIDNEYS

The kidneys are two organs or glands, each about the size of one's fist. They are suspended in the back, on the rear wall of the abdomen. They hang loosely near the spinal column, suspended by a ligament. Their purpose is to filter the water in the body as it is passed through them by the blood stream.

Small as they are, they filter about 5,500 gallons of water a year. Although they filter about 4 gallons of water every day, only 2 to 4 pints a day is passed out as waste through the bladder, as urine. The rest of the water is re-circulated throughout the system, by the blood stream.

Every drop of liquid which enters our system must pass through the kidneys to be filtered. The blood consists of about 3/5ths water. In other words, 3 quarts out of the total 5 quarts of blood in the body is water. Irrespective of how much liquid we drink, the water content of the blood never changes. All the excess of the water we drink over and above the 3 quarts contained in the blood, is stored in the muscles and in the liver. However, every drop of water in the system is constantly passed through the kidneys for filtering.

Our Creator very evidently knew how much trouble He would have with us in our efforts to avoid "Becoming Younger". He made our body, and particularly the most vital and important parts of our body so elastic, that we could continue to live or to exist, for a while at least, in spite of ourselves.

Consider the kidneys as just one example. They are a truly miraculous filtering apparatus. They consist of more than 30 **billion** cells. These cells are grouped into clusters of filter coils. Each filter coil is no larger than a speck of dust, yet it is composed of about 15,000 cells. If you can visualize anything so microscopic and marvelous, you can realize what a wonderful and delicate organ we have which protects us day and night, as long as we live, from our careless appetites and habits.

All drugs and alcoholic beverages are exceedingly harmful to the kidneys, irrespective of the temporary benefits which may be derived by any other part of the body. Beer is probably the most destructive liquid which we can put into our system. I have examined a tremendous number of kidneys at autopsies which I have been able to

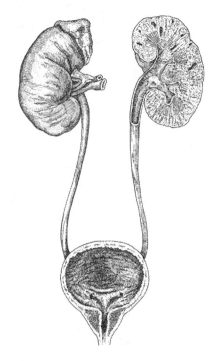

attend, and I could invariably determine correctly the alcoholic habits of the deceased. I found that beer disintegrated kidneys very fast. In England, where the workingman considers beer and ale his heritage, kidney ailments are the most outstanding afflictions. In the United States, where breweries are on a rampage with their beer advertisements to lure the uninformed and the gullible, kidney ailments are increasing daily. In the brief span of only 10 years, the alcoholic output jumped from less than 350 million gallons, to more than **1 billion 176 million gallons**.

It is only because of the tremendous number of cells in the kidneys, and their miraculous efficiency, that so many people are able to struggle through a few score years of life, in spite of the destructive liquids which they pour into their system.

"Soft drinks" are nearly always sweetened with sugar. The combination causes alcohol to form in the body, and this must go through the kidneys for filtering. The damage to children, adolescents and young people, no less than to older people, from the use of such beverages, is almost unbelievable. The insidious part of this damage is that it does not become manifest immediately. It gives a false "uplift" temporarily, but the subsequent let-down, hours or days afterwards, is rarely if ever attributed to the use of these beverages.

The water in the human system is one element whose importance surpasses that of all the other elements, except oxygen in the air.

Youthfulness in man and woman is determined mainly by the fluidity of its vitality. Vitality must flow constantly and freely through the entire system. This vitality is dependent on the purity and fluidity of the blood stream and the lymph which in their very nature hinges on the **quality** of the water in the body.

Water that is not constantly replenished becomes stagnant and polluted. In the body, such stagnation results in sickness and disease and is manifested as body odor, or a pale, sallow or ashen complexion. This means premature aging.

The abundant use of fresh raw vegetable and fruit juices furnish the body with the very finest quality of **organic** water obtainable. If we drink enough of these juices, we need hardly ever drink any water. I personally do not drink a glass of water a year except the hot water and lemon juice which I drink every morning upon arising. BUT I drink as much of the fresh vegetable and fruit juices as I can conveniently take. I find that the lemon juice in hot water helps wonderfully to flush the liver and the kidneys. On the other hand I have found that by drinking it cold it helps to stimulate the peristalsis of the intestines and frequently helps the early morning elimination.

Have you ever wondered why so many liver and kidney pills are advertised so extensively? It is because it is a known fact that liver and kidney troubles and ailments are on the increase. The reason is the increased consumption of beverages and foods which damage these organs, on the one hand, and on the other hand, insufficient education on the value and benefits of the fresh raw vegetable juices.

May I suggest, as good educational reading on the subject, that you obtain a copy of the book FRESH VEGETABLE AND FRUIT JUICES, What's Missing In Your Body?

A lifetime of study and research has gone into compiling it. You will find listed in it the juices most beneficial and helpful, and the best way to extract them. Innumerable people have written to me saying that this book has been a means to help them rejuvenate, to "Become Younger".

DRINKING WATER, OTHER VIOLATIONS

Under federal law, all public water systems must meet minimum health standards. A new report shows these instances of violations of the Safe Drinking Water Act:

State	Excessive contaminants violations	Monitoring, reporting violations
Alabama	55	327
Alaska	233	19,119
Arizona	405	14,886
Arkansas	101	245
California	894	3,396
Colorado	90	782
Connecticut	234	565
Delaware	107	5
D.C.	0	2
Florida	521	5,250
Georgia	169	746
Hawaii	34	40
Idaho	464	1,342
Illinois	730	2,514
Indiana	42	917
Iowa	264	2,359
Kansas	178	291
Kentucky	130	1,461
Louisiana	529	162
Maine	65	154
Maryland	68	264
Massachusetts	113	257
Michigan	155	241
Minnesota	59	469
Missouri	422	850
Mississippi	339	835
Montana	113	1,136
Nebraska	377	70
Nevada	24	367
New York	406	6,174
New Jersey	215	2,819
New Hampshire	335	382
New Mexico	131	473
North Carolina	338	20,054
North Dakota	84	154
Ohio	576	3,085
Oklahoma	532	855
Oregon	309	1,521
Pennsylvania	459	12,897
Rhode Island	29	27
South Carolina	91	1,279
South Dakota	306	1,204
Tennessee	42	250
Texas	822	2,329
Utah	115	613
Vermont	272	892
Virginia	496	1,464
Washington	1,474	7,993
West Virginia	92	817
Wisconsin	164	433
Wyoming	54	482

Source: Natural Resources Defense Council

USA Today 9/27/93

HOW DID YOUR STATE RANK IN EPA VIOLATIONS?

Chapter 28
HOW SAFE IS YOUR DRINKING WATER?

The Centers for Disease Control recorded twenty six thousand microscopically spread water born illnesses between 1986 and 1988. Officials believe this to be a mere fraction of the real total since all outbreaks are not accurately noted and reported. According to U.S. News and World Report, "water-born illness is almost certainly on the rise." In 1994 the government reported more than 400,000 cases of people becoming ill due to impure city water services.

Chemical treatment procedures are of equal concern. The long term affect of chlorine has serious complications. After having been combined with water and organic material (such as fertilizer and decaying leaves) it produces by-products, many of which have proven to be carcinogenic in animals.

Kenneth Cantor and his colleagues from the National Cancer Institute studied three thousand patients recently diagnosed with bladder cancer. Their findings were that chlorinated water may as much as doubled the risk of the illness. In Cantor's words "When you consider the widespread exposure, the increase in risk is potentially tens of thousands of cases a year." Chlorine is but one of many chemicals used in treatment plants, the combination of their long-term carcinogenic affect should concern us all. We can't even be assured that all microbes will be destroyed because unfortunately many have become chemically resistant.

The filtering procedures used today in our treatment plants are inferior as well. Many microbes are just too minute to be filtered out. It is essential that the correct size filter, which is one that captures all particles of one micron or larger, be used.

What about bacteria?

Cryptosporidium is a chlorine resistant protozoan and ranges from between four to six microns in size. It is the parasite from which one hundred people died and thousands became ill in Milwaukee in 1993. This was not the first outbreak or the worst, and it will most certainly not be the last. The eggs of the Cryptosporidium parasite hatch in the human digestive tract. Symptoms includes severe diarrhea, cramps, vomiting, fever, and in certain cases death.

This particular parasite infiltrates our water supply by way of animal and human sewage. The Associated Press reports that according to antibody tests, half the population of the United States has been affected at one time or another.

Dr. Hubert Dupont is the chairman of the Infectious Disease Department at the University of Texas Medical School in Houston. He explains that in this country as much as twenty five percent of the samples collected from "treated water" have had this organism, and that in developing countries the infection rates have soared as high as ninety percent.

To those people whose immune systems have been seriously compromised, the introduction of such a parasite into their intestinal tract has proved devastating and deadly. People, for instance who are HIV positive or have full blown AIDS would be especially vulnerable to such water born diseases as cryptosporidium.

It is obvious that the E.P.A. has need to establish a more precise and deliberate way in which these parasites can be removed from our water supply. They are most commonly found in "surface water" and because many water treatment plants draw from "surface water", as does Lake Michigan for instance, they are required to file monthly operating reports with the Department of Natural Resources. This procedure does not however include any state or federally regulated health standard to be met in regards to the existence of cryptosporidium in drinking water.

Presently the Environmental Protection Agency's information on the transmittal or the treatment of this specific parasite is inadequate. To date, the "federal surface water treatment regulation" doesn't even include any information on cryptosporidium.

It is interesting to note that killing this protozoan is simple, it dies at two hundred and twelve degrees fahrenheit, as do bacteria viruses and cysts.

Distilled water will exterminate all parasitical life at one hundred and eighty five degrees fahrenheit (before it even reaches boiling). This is because distilling creates steam. When the steam rises it leaves the bacteria that it has killed behind. Chemicals and other pollutants are removed as well and what remains is simply clean, safe water. Interestingly enough it's not uncommon that many people remain relatively unconcerned about the quality of something they could not live more than three days without.

The truth is that for optimum efficiency the human body is emphatically dependent on fresh, clean water. Without enough of it your chemical, biological and mechanical functions will all suffer. The entire human body consists of seventy percent water and every five to ten days it is replaced completely. Everything from brain cells to muscle tone, daily digestion, heart, liver, and breathing functions to dry skin and kidney activity is in need of generous daily amounts of pure, uncontaminated water.

Want a little added encouragement? For those of you who are dieting or working diligently to maintain healthy weight, water is imperative. Drinking eight to twelve 8-ounce glasses of distilled water a day raises and maintains your metabolism in "optimum" working order! Drink up!

Chapter 29

DR. WALKER'S PROGRAM
TO A HEALTHIER MORE VIBRANT LIFE

Raw vegetable and fruit juices offer all the live enzymes and detoxicating qualities needed to keep our bodies strong, healthy and able to combat the many enemies of contamination and pollution in the world today. Our immune systems are kept at their peak when we consume "raw" vegetable and fruit juices on a daily basis. Vegetable juices are the "builders" of the body, while fruit juices are the "cleansers". Every cell, gland and organ benefits from pure, natural form of nutrition. It is comforting to realize that by drinking raw vegetable and fruit juices every day, our diet is complete in all the vitamins and minerals it needs to remain younger, stronger and healthier.

"Fresh Vegetable and Fruit Juices" by Dr. N. W. Walker was written to better explain and emphasize the procedures and specific benefits of juicing. Raw carrot juice for instance is rich in Vitamins A, B, B, C, D, E, and K. Properly prepared raw carrot juice aids digestion and is valuable in the maintenance of the bone structure that supports our entire body, including the teeth. Even intestinal and liver diseases are sometimes due to the lack of certain vitamins and minerals found in raw carrot juice. Endive juice contains elements essential to the optic systems while the cucumber juice offers the best of diuretic qualities. The list goes on.

It is well worth one's time to study the benefits derived from "fresh raw" juices. Actually, it's worth far more than your time . . . after all, this is your health and your life. Take control, feel better, look younger, and enjoy your life more completely. You are worth it!

Keep the colon clean. The health of your colon can be an indicator of your health. Laxatives are not healthy and certainly not the proper answer to constipation. Raw vegetable salads, fresh fruits, legumes and unprocessed grains along with plenty of distilled water will keep your colon regular and healthy. "Colonic Irrigations" once or twice a year, along with enemas done at home, offer an optimum way in which to insure a clean and active, healthy intestinal track. Being "regular" is having a bowel movement at least once a day, though often times two or three movements a day is ideal. The elimination of red meat and all processed foods from the diet is equally important. A well cleansed colon in perfect working order is absolutely essential for a long, productive and active life. It is important to note that when the colon is healthy, and not blocked, you are avoiding innumerable ailments. Because the colon is a natural breeding ground for pathogenic bacteria, it is essential that we prevent a toxic condition from developing in the colon. By maintaining a proper and clean environment for the "good bacteria" we avoid the "bad bacteria" which is dangerous and disease producing.

Drink PURE water. The body is dependent on fresh, clean water. The minerals, bacteria, and commercial additives in inorganic water (i.e. tap, spring, well water, etc.) are inorganic and cannot be utilized by the body. The vitamins and minerals within vegetables and fruits and their juices are organic and therefore beneficial to your health. Distilled water is in reality steam that has condensed back into water. Bacteria, parasites (including Cryptosporidium parvum that is so devastating to those in ill health) is destroyed by the distillation process. Some authorities believe that distilled water acts like a "sponge" and assits the body in eliminating toxins, etc. through the body's normal elimination processes. Drink plenty of vegetable and fruit juices and distilled water.

Regular exercise. It keeps our hearts healthy, our blood pressure intact, our respiratory systems strong, and our metabolism balanced. Walking is the best exercise you can do. It can burn calories and tone muscles. In addition to weight control, exercise strengthens the immune system, relieves stress, and because of the release of endorphins, lifts your spirits. Recent medical research has found that during exercise the body releases several different chemicals, some of which have been found to deter cancer. A 30-minute walk every day is truly beneficial to your health. Also, bear in mind that the body needs sufficient rest and sleep to function at its' best.

Control your weight. Weight control is a very real and all to common problem among Americans today. Carrying an excess amount of weight dramatically affects the state of ones overall health. High blood pressure, clogged arteries and fatigue are only a few reasons why maintaining a healthy weight is so imperative. A long and healthy life cannot be achieved when the body is forced to deal with such a myriad of dilemmas. Weight control need not even be an issue if we simply restrict our food consumption to salads composed of raw vegetables and fruits, drink their juices and distilled water. You will feel much healthier and your vitality will increase, when all red meats, fats, commercial sugars and starches are eliminated from the diet.

The elimination of unhealthy products. Some of the most harmful food products consumed today include processed sugars, harmful fats, cow's milk and soft drinks. Because the human body does not tolerate, and in many cases, is damaged from the consumption of such products, one would be wise to consider not ingesting them. This elimination may very well in and of itself, better insure a longer and healthier life. The pancreas, for instance, is both overworked and subject to disturbing reactions when we consume sugar. When the body processes meat it produces a great deal of uric acid. The muscles absorb much of what should be expelled through the eliminative system and what sometimes occurs is the manifestation of various conditions such as rheumatism, neuritis and sciatic. It is self-preserving not to tempt bad health with bad food choices.

Alcohol and tobacco products are carcinogenic, organ damaging and life threatening to all who imbibe. Though these habits remain widespread throughout our world today, few would argue of their obvious dangers to our health and to the negative effect on the very length of life itself. To live longer, healthier and with vitality, we should eliminate all detrimental products from our lives.

Other vital nutrients that play important defense roles in your health include plentiful amounts of Vitamin C, raw onions and garlic. They offer strong immune boosting qualities, act as an excellent cleansing agents, are readily available, and should be taken advantage of on a regular basis. Ideally we would all grow our own food in our own healthy soil. But this of course, is not an option for the majority of our population. What is possible is selecting the best of all foods that you can possibly find.

Last, but not least, is our spiritual and emotional health. Stress, anger, resentment, the need to "get even" are all negative emotions and can play havoc with our physical health. Heart attacks, strokes and nervous disorders are only a few of the conditions associated with such a negative life-style. The opposite of negativism is optimism. Laughter, spiritual strength, the ability to forgive and forget, to deal with our every day problems with an attitude of solving them is essential to keep the glands in our body working together. Our physical health is dependent upon a calm, serene mental attitude.

Self-preservation utilizes wisdom. The knowledge and application of defensive procedures can do much to protect and lengthen our lives. For instance, it is as wise to always wear a seatbelt as it is to avoid preservatives and pollutants whenever possible. Adopting and exchanging unhealthy habits to healthy habits is as easy as eating smaller meals, eating them more frequently, and chewing ones' food for a longer period of time are changes your entire digestive system will thank you for. Utilize your wisdom, it will benefit you greatly in your quest to live a long and vibrant life.

CONCLUSION

For centuries, millions of people have been drinking whatever water was available and did not instantly perish by doing so.

Nevertheless, there is no telling how many millions of people have suffered untold misery and a premature death by the clogging up of veins and arteries. The accumulation of inorganic calcium over a lifetime, ingested by their consumption of Natural Water, no doubt went undiagnosed.

Until recently I, too, drank whatever water was available, without a thought about the calcium danger lurking in such a liquid.

Of course for a great many years I have been drinking fresh raw vegetable and fruit juices, daily. These consisted of the finest inherent Naturally Distilled Water, replete with organic mineral elements. I feel I can justly attribute my present Vibrant Health, energy, vigor and vitality to the ample drinking of these juices.

Thus, several years ago I was led to find many new discoveries and recently I recognized the danger which is lurking in Natural waters in which are mineral elements incompatible for use by the cells of the body, and with which the body, today, should not be afflicted. It is likely, because the human body cannot tolerate these types of minerals, that they may eventually cause grievous harm.

Thereupon I was led to thoroughly investigate the problem, and I discovered the solution, namely, not to use Natural Waters but to use

Steam Distilled Water for drinking and for the preparation of foods. This is exactly what we, in my family, have been doing with much apparent benefit.

In publishing this dissertation on the subject of Distilled Water, there is neither purpose nor design on my part to instill fear in anybody's mind, nor to influence people to practice rigidly what I have expounded in this book.

You are a free moral agent and the choice of Natural or Distilled Water is yours only.

After all it is your life with which YOU are concerned. YOU ALONE can choose and practice or not, that which can develop either health or sickness, a long, happy, energetic, vitally interesting life, or, on the contrary, a mere state of tolerant existence for a few brief years culminating in a premature, useless old age.

The gift of health and of an abundant life is our heritage, if we wish to claim it and practice it.

ADDENDUM

WHAT AUTHORITATIVE SOURCES ARE TELLING US ABOUT THE WATER WE DRINK

Over the past 20 years America's drinking water problems have continued to multiply. All the new laws - all the public disclosures have not cleaned up our water.

We found hundreds of articles, written by authoritative persons for our government, by university research departments and reporters in the public domain. Newspapers, magazines, as well as television and radio programs have been reporting stories of deaths and illness caused from citizens drinking bacteria infested water from our so-called 'safe water systems'.

Perhaps you may be interested in reading a brief summary of reference material we uncovered.

- Federal Government officials had "reports about CRYPTOSPORIDIUM parasites as early as 1974 - when a 3-year-old girl became ill in Tennessee."

The Washington Post, 9/26/1993

- A similar outbreak was reported in Carrollton, Georgia when 13,000 people became ill with a similar "bug".

  The Washington Post, 9/26/1993

- In 1987 the EPA passed the Safe Drinking Water Act," but did NOT require testing or treatment for Cryptosporidium even though EPA said the parasite was found in virtually all surface waters", and was responsible for illness around the world and could be fatal for those with immune problems.

  The Washington Post, 9/26/1993

- More than 1 in 5 Americans drink tap water polluted with feces, radiation or other contaminates . . . "Nearly 1,000 deaths occur each year and at least 400,000 cases of waterborne illnesses may be attributed to contaminated water".

  The New York Times, 6/2/1995

- "The General Accounting Office (GOA) estimates that 66% of violations under the Safe Drinking Water Acts are NOT reported".

  USA Today, 7/28/1994

- The GOA also reported that "90% of the major water utilities have failed to install post-World War I technologies to remove contaminants and said millions of Americans are drinking water that does not meet federal standards" . . . The report also stated that although Chlorine is widely used to disinfect water, the report continued with the fact that water is not being treated against cancer-linked by-products formed by the reaction of Chlorine to organic materials.

  The Orlando Sentinel, 3/15/1994

- "120 million Americans may be needlessly exposed to unhealthy drinking water. In 1991-92, 43% of all water supplies violated federal health standards. Violations totalled over 250,000 affecting more than 900,000 persons who became ill - and possibly 900 deaths. State and federal regulators acted on just 3,900 of these violations".

  USA Today, 9/27/93

- In 1993 the EPA enacted new guidelines for utility companies to comply with regarding tighter limits. Cryptosporidium was NOT included in these new guidelines. The EPA did state that in the future it could impose additional requirements if current requirements are inadequate to control Cryptosporidium.

WQA Newsletter, April/May 1993

- Government officials recommend that people with weakened immune systems boil their water to avoid a dangerous parasitic illness, a precaution that officials had warned Southern Nevada physicians treating AIDS patients a year earlier. Weakened immune systems can include organ transplant patients and those receiving cancer treatment.

Las Vegas Review-Journal, 6/16/1995

- The 1993 outbreak of parasitic contamination of the water supply left more than 200,000 feeling the effects. They experienced severe diarrhea, nausea, stomach cramps and other digestive distress. More than 100 people died. Yet, according to Ms. Browner, head of the EPA, which sets standards for drinking water standards, Milwaukee treatment plants were not in violation of EPA standards. Those "most at risk" of the parasite are those with weakened immune systems, infants and elderly, patients on chemotherapy and especially with HIV. **DATELINE, 9/1994**

- Among contaminants within our water supply systems are such contaminants as: lead, zinc, selenium, uranium, molybdenum, silver, nickel, mercury, cadmium, cobalt, tin, chrome, arsenic, barium, lithium, boron, silicon, aluminum and sulphur to name only a few. Even though our bodies need some of the items mentioned - these are inorganic. Our bodies can only utilize such materials as are found in their organic state (which you can only get from the food you eat).

Various Sources

- The eliminative system of the body (kidneys, intestines, pores of the skin, etc.) eliminate a portion of the inorganic materials. Many of the medical professionals believe that these inorganic minerals accumulate in our bodies. It is logical to assume that the materials not expelled from the body will accumulate in various parts of the body and the accumulative could be detrimental to our health and well-being in the form of arthritis and hardening of the arteries.

- According to many professionals it is best to drink "pure" water. Pure water is usually considered to be either "filtered", "reverse osmosis" or "distilled" water.

- Carbon "Filtered" water must have an absolute rating of ONE MICRON to trap the parasites - however, it does not kill them, therefore the filters can be a breeding ground for such parasites.

- "Reverse Osmosis" also will remove chemicals, minerals, and TRAP the parasites - but does not kill them. It is extremely important to follow the manufacturers guidelines in installation and maintenance.

- "Distilled" Water is pure water. Since the Cryptosporidium parasite can be killed by heating water to 185^OF. for 5 minutes - distilling your water kills the parasites, viruses, cysts, as well as removing all chemicals and minerals.

- When a city or town has pollution within their water systems, one of the first "news alerts" the officials issue is BOIL YOUR WATER. By using distilled water you have already removed the danger - BEFORE the officials notify you that the water is contaminated.

- There are some studies by professionals that distilled water will assist the body in disposing of accumulated inorganic minerals and chemicals.

A SUMMARY OF REFERENCE MATERIAL

Governmental and Environmental Groups. . .

- The Environmental Protection Agency (EPA), the Center for Disease Control and Prevention (CDC) plus two reports from the Natural Resources Defense Council & Environmentalist Working Group all state that our drinking tap water could not only be dangerous, but possibly fatal for up to six million Americans with weakened immune systems.

- The EWG (Environmental Working Group) report fecal coliform bacteria in 1,172 water systems, lead in 2,551 systems, and radioactive materials (such as radon) in 325 systems.

- AND the government is actually considering weakening the Safe Water Drinking Act.

Water and Aging . . .

- Insufficient water intake interferes with our physical performance and our mental health - the average person loses 75% of their kidney function by the age of 70.

- Our bodies are composed of 66% water - however this percentage of water tends to drop as we grow older. Chronic dehydration affects most of the elderly and without adequate water intake there is a build-up of toxic and inorganic debris within the body.

Medical . . .

- Researchers and scientists began piecing together evidence on Chlorine's hazards almost three years ago and have concluded that cancer, infertility and animal reproductive abnormalities are caused by synthetic chemicals - most of them chlorine based - whose molecular structure resemble human estrogens.

- The eight- year-old son of a medical doctor had allergic reaction which progressed into severe asthma. The boy was given eight 8-ounce glasses of water per day and a balanced diet. In four days his symptoms had improved so much, he stopped medication and in one month he was entirely normal.

Health . . .

- A 1986 EPA study estimated that more than 40 million Americans drink water containing excessive lead levels.

- In fiscal year 1990, 1 in 5 water suppliers violated health standards or did NOT adequately test drinking water - the EPA took enforcement against only a few of the chronic offenders.

- Water is a great weight control measure. Drink a lot between meals, you will be less hungry and water will increase your metabolism.

- Kidney dialysis machines use only distilled water - because chemicals in public water supplies (including Chlorine and Fluorides) have adverse affects on kidney patients.

- Chlorine is so potent, it is transported in rubberized tanks. It is used primarily for disinfecting, fumigating and bleaching.

- The U.S. Navy makes distilled water from sea water. (Can you imagine how much water they would have to store on-board if they were not self-contained with their own water purification system?)

- Catalina Island (off the Southern Coast of California) supplies their entire population and tourism industry with pure water from its own reverse osmosis system.

- Virtually all laboratory experiments are conducted with distilled water - to avoid contaminants that are in our public water systems.

- Some studies link bladder cancer with the chlorinated water.

- Lead in our public water systems impairs our children's mental development and attention span.

- Some naturopathic physicians, nutritionists, chiropractors, etc. suggest that you consume sufficient "pure" water to equal one-half your weight in ounces. Accordingly, a person weighing 120 pounds should consume 60 ounces of "pure" water. Some of this "pure" water can be supplied by the fruits and vegetables (including their juices) which you eat every day. This is minimum - if you exercise when it is hot, low humidity, and/or overweight for your gender. . . increase your daily intake of water.

- Although distilled water is "pure" - no chemicals, minerals, etc. It is well to consider and realize the body CANNOT utilize man-made chemicals and minerals. They should come from the fruits and vegetables we eat each day. All fruits and vegetables contain varying amounts of the minerals and vitamins the body needs and they are organic (made by nature).

Do you know THE MAGIC OF OUR WATER?
- At 32° Fahrenheit, ground level water freezes - yet at high altitude it remains a liquid until the temperature drops below MINUS 10° Fahrenheit.

- Ice floats on top because water becomes lighter when it turns into a solid. . . NO other substance does that.

- Clear water is chemically neutral. . . yet water is the BEST solvent known and contains almost ALL other substances dissolved, remaining neither acidic or alkaline.

- IF the Gulf Stream did not contain an unbelievable amount of heat energy and release it along the European Coast - Europe would be colder than Hudson Bay, Canada.

INDEX

FRESH VEGETABLE AND FRUIT JUICES
What's Missing In Your Body?*
By N. W. Walker, D. Sc.

New, Revised and Enlarged Edition
If we are well, we should drink Juices to keep well. If there is anything the matter with us, then we certainly should drink Juices, and plenty of them, every day. What Juices to drink? Why? How can Juices be made, to extract ALL the Vitamins and Mineral elements contained in vegetables and fruits? This book points out in masterly and convincing manner WHICH Juices to use — and why.

This is the only book we have ever found that contains authoritative information on vegetable juices and JUICE THERAPY based on more than 25 years of research and first hand experience.

Thousands upon thousands of copies of this book have been bought the world over — because people want dependable and authoritative information on vegetable juices.

This book describes 150 ailments so the layman can understand their cause and origin, and do something about them. Juices and their combinations are indicated which have given consistently beneficial results. Learn how to combine your juices, and in what proportions.

* Edited and Revised. 1995

Fresh Vegetables And Fruit Juices

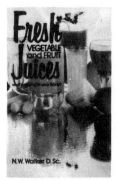

In FRESH VEGETABLES AND FRUIT JUICES, R. D. Pope, M.D., writes–"Dr. Walker has, for the first time in history, written a complete guide of the Therapeutic uses of our more common, every-day vegetables when taken in the form of fresh, raw juices. It will be of considerable help to those who wish to derive the utmost benefit from the natural foods which God created for the nourishment of Man." Dr. Walker categorically lists vegetable juices, explains their elements, and in cooperation with Doctor Pope, provides suggestions for effective treatment of special ailments.

Colon Health: The Key To A Vibrant Life

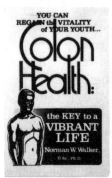

In COLON HEALTH Dr. Walker will take this forgotten part of your body and focus your full attention on it–and you'll never again take it for granted! This books shows how every organ, gland and cell in the body is affected by the condition of the large intestine–the colon. COLON HEALTH answers such questions as: Are cathartics and laxatives dangerous? Can colon care prevent heart attack?–Is your eyesight affected by the condition of your colon?–What are the ghastly results of a colostomy?

Vegetarian Guide To Diet And Salad

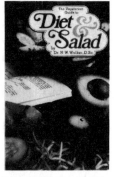

The pitfalls of overindulgence in certain food elements, especially oil and sugar, have been well documented. Dr. Walker offers in his book DIET & SALAD both a cook book and a nutritional guide that belongs in every homemaker's kitchen. In it he supports current medical research about the harmful effects of milk–"It is generally assumed that cow's milk is one of our mòst perfect foods... Milk is the most mucus forming food in the human dietary, and it is the most insidious cause of colds, flu, bronchial troubles, asthma, hay fever, pneumonia, and sinus trouble... cow's milk was never intended for a human infant."

Water Can Undermine Your Health

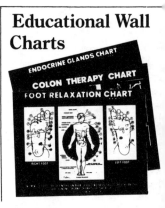

Dr. Walker sees water pollution as a cause of arthritis, varicose veins, cancer, and even heart attacks–a major problem in virtually every community in the country. His treatment of water pollution is revealing, comprehensive, and scientific. His findings, and his recommendations for corrective action, offer new hope.

Educational Wall Charts

ENDOCRINE GLANDS CHART
COLON THERAPY CHART
FOOT RELAXATION CHART

RIGHT FOOT   LEFT FOOT